A Breast Cancer Guide for Spouses, Partners, Friends, and Family

This practical, science-based book focuses on helping partners, family, and friends understand breast cancer. It guides them in how to provide the best emotional and practical support when helping someone with breast cancer to cope, recover, and thrive, while maintaining their own physical and psychological health.

The authors translate psychological evidence into concrete, practical advice for caregivers, validated through their first-hand experience. It also suggests ways to help someone with breast cancer make the best decisions in consultation with oncology professionals. The authors draw on well-established psychological principles relevant to social attitudes, how decisions are made, good communication skills, empathy, and how to better understand the ideas and worries experienced by women who have, or may have, breast cancer and those close to them. Each chapter includes "How you can Help" sections that give specific and concrete suggestions, as well as a chapter summary of the main points along with recommendations and additional resources.

It is essential reading for all those who want to help and support a loved one with breast cancer. It is also useful for training healthcare professionals in how to support partners.

Stephen N. Haynes obtained his PhD at the University of Colorado, USA and is Emeritus Professor of Psychology at the University of Hawai'i at Mānoa, USA. Dr. Haynes has published widely in the areas of psychological assessment and psychopathology. His wife was diagnosed with breast cancer and she had experienced two 3D mammograms, a biopsy, three lumpectomies, a mastectomy, months of chemotherapy, weeks of radiation therapy, and many treatment side effects.

Luanna H. Meyer, PhD, was professor of education in the USA at the Universities of Hawai'i and Minnesota, Syracuse University, and in New Zealand at Massey University and Victoria University, where she is Professor Emerita. She has published widely. Her treatment for triple-negative breast cancer included chemotherapy, bilateral mastectomy, and breast reconstruction.

Ian M. Evans obtained his PhD at the Institute of Psychiatry, London, UK. He has taught clinical psychology in the USA at universities in Hawai'i, and Binghamton, and Waikato and Massey in New Zealand. His work includes the emotional development of children and the practice of behavioral psychotherapy. He is a Fellow of The Royal Society of New Zealand.

A Breast Cancer Guide for Spouses, Partners, Friends, and Family

Using Psychology to Support
Those We Care About

Stephen N. Haynes
Luanna H. Meyer, and
Ian M. Evans

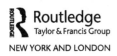

Routledge
Taylor & Francis Group

NEW YORK AND LONDON

Cover image: Megumi, two years before, during, and two years after breast cancer treatments, © Supplied by author

First published 2022
by Routledge
605 Third Avenue, New York, NY 10158
and by Routledge
2 Park Square, Milton Park, Abingdon, Oxon, OX14 4RN
Routledge is an imprint of the Taylor & Francis Group, an informa business

Library of Congress Cataloguing-in-Publication Data
Names: Haynes, Stephen N., 1944- author. | Meyer, Luanna H., 1945- author. | Evans, Ian M., 1944- author.
Title: A breast cancer guide for spouses, partners, friends, and family : using psychology to support those we care about / Stephen N. Haynes, Luanna H. Meyer and Ian M. Evans.
Description: New York, NY : Routledge, 2022. | Includes bibliographical references and index. |
Identifiers: LCCN 2021037661 (print) | LCCN 2021037662 (ebook) | ISBN 9781032046495 (paperback) | ISBN 9781032046501 (hardback) | ISBN 9781003194088 (ebook)
Subjects: LCSH: Breast--Cancer--Patients. | Breast--Cancer--Patients--Family relationships. | Breast--Cancer--Patients--Psychological aspects.
Classification: LCC RC280.B8 H3985 2022 (print) | LCC RC280.B8 (ebook) | DDC 616.99/449--dc23
LC record available at https://lccn.loc.gov/2021037661
LC ebook record available at https://lccn.loc.gov/2021037662

ISBN: 978-1-032-04650-1 (hbk)
ISBN: 978-1-032-04649-5 (pbk)
ISBN: 978-1-003-19408-8 (ebk)

DOI: 10.4324/9781003194088

Typeset in Bembo
by MPS Limited, Dehradun

SNH: To Megumi and her radiation, therapy, and oncology teams

LHM: In memory of my sister Bonnie Meyer Jensen, 1947–1993

IME: To the medical staff of Kaiser Permanente, Hawai'i

Contents

Acknowledgments

Many friends and colleagues have contributed their expertise and wisdom to this book, both directly and indirectly, however there are some especially important people whom we would like to thank.

First, we sought and received formal technical reviews and advice from two leading experts, for whose contribution we are enormously grateful:

Keola K. Beale, MD, is a clinical oncologist at Kaiser Permanente in Honolulu, Hawai'i. He is Board Certified in Hematology and in Medical Oncology. His MD is from the University of California at San Francisco Medical School. He states that "personal experience inspired me to focus on oncology. For me, this specialty is the perfect blend of tremendously interesting science and amazing patients." Dr. Beale provided a technical review of an early draft of this book and helped to correct any errors or misunderstandings of medical details on our part. He also affirms in his bio he strives "every day to provide the best care that I can and to treat every patient as I would treat my own loved one," and we have personal experience that that is true.

Alicia K. Matthews, PhD, is Professor, Department of Population Health Nursing Science and Associate Dean for Equity and Inclusion in the College of Nursing, University of Illinois at Chicago. As we know well, her doctoral training was in clinical psychology at the State University of New York at Binghamton. She is widely acclaimed nationally and internationally for her research and experience in examining determinants of cancer-related health disparities with a focus on racial/ethnic minorities and other underserved populations. Dr. Matthews provided detailed and invaluable commentary on our efforts to make this book beneficial to the widest possible range of readership.

Second, significant others have provided input, guidance from their personal and sometimes painful life experiences, and encouragement for our attempt to provide a guide that would be helpful, readable, and insightful. They brought stories, wisdom, grammatical niceties, insightful suggestions, "what?!" questions, and even words of reinforcement. In alphabetical order only, these are the critical friends who have helped us so well: *Robert Jensen, Joseph Laturnau, Lori Lipari-Jordan, Gerald Mager, Charles Mueller, and Christine Nelson.* Mahalo nui mākou and aloha to all of you. We are so fortunate to have had your input and the generosity of your thoughts.

Stephen, Luanna, and Ian
Honolulu, Hawaii, November 2021

Preface

Breast cancer affects millions of women and can have devastating impact on many aspects of a woman's life. It can also affect her husband, wife, partner, friends, siblings, children, parents, grandchildren, colleagues, and grandparents. Breast cancer can be especially stressful for persons who are intimately involved in helping her with the difficult treatment and recovery phases of breast cancer. Research from psychology and behavioral medicine tells us that emotional and practical support from those who care about a woman with breast cancer can strengthen her quality of life and promote recovery.

You are probably reading this Guide because you want to know how to best support the woman you care about who is facing breast cancer, and it can be difficult to know what to say or do and what not to say and do. This Guide offers many suggestions for ways you can help her. We encourage you to pick those that feel right for you and her.

The emotional effects of breast cancer on you can be especially profound when you are an important caregiver for her. Breast cancer can affect your relationship, how and what the two of you talk about, your children's sense of well-being, how often you visit with friends and family members, your recreational and leisure activities, what you eat, and your emotional and physical health. Thus, this Guide also emphasizes the importance of maintaining your own emotional and physical health while you are helping her cope with this destabilizing and life-threatening disease.

We suggest many principles for caregiving throughout the Guide. Because people differ in the level and type of support they prefer, one of the most important suggestions we make is to avoid assuming that you know what is best for her – *offer your support and ask her what would be most helpful*. We also offer suggestions about practical ways you can help, such as arranging transportation to treatment sessions, helping out with daily tasks when she is fatigued, helping her communicate with her oncology team, how to do home injections, and what to say about her breast cancer to children, family, and friends.

Many of the effects of breast cancer depend on the type and severity of the cancer. This is not a medically oriented book, but we do provide basic information about the types of breast cancer and its severity, such as stage of the cancer, so as to give you some background and help you understand all aspects of her treatment. At the end of each chapter we provide additional sources that contain science-based information about breast cancer, its treatments, and ways to support a woman with breast cancer.

Although parts of this Guide would be informative for her, it is not directed at the breast cancer patient, and it does not make treatment recommendations. Those are shared decisions made by her oncology team and her. She makes the ultimate decision about her treatments, and we suggest ways that you can help her consider various potential decisions.

This Guide discusses many aspects of breast cancer, its treatment, and how breast cancer and its treatments can affect her, you, and others, both physically and mentally. We inform you about the effects of breast cancer and its treatments so that you can better understand her experience and the many ways you can support her while maintaining your own health. We draw on well-established psychological principles, not just about feelings but also issues relating to judgment and social attitudes, how decisions are made and influenced, good communication skills, empathy, and how to better understand the ideas and worries that any children in the family may have.

Separate chapters in the Guide discuss basic information about breast cancer and its treatments; the many decisions that must be made during the diagnosis and treatment of breast cancer; how breast cancer is detected, diagnosed, and monitored; biopsies and genetic testing; lumpectomies and breast-conserving surgery; chemotherapy; radiation treatment; mastectomies; breast reconstruction; and the development of a treatment summary and survivorship care plan in coordination with her oncology team. We also cover how to talk to family and friends; how to talk to and involve children; metastatic breast cancer; and ways to cope with stress and stay healthy. At the end of each chapter we present a summary of the main points and recommendations.

We emphasize a science-based approach, respect for cultural and spiritual values, and how your understanding about breast cancer treatments can support a woman with breast cancer. There are thousands of scientific reports that could be cited, but at the end of each chapter we have identified what we judge to be particularly useful, authoritative, and up-to-date books, research articles, and websites for additional information. There are many types of cancer other than breast cancer and men can also have breast cancer. Although many of the recommendations are relevant for anyone who wants to support a person with a chronic disease, this Guide is written for supporters of women with breast cancer. We also recognize that not all those with breast cancer may identify as female, though for the purposes of ease we have used the gender binary pronouns of she/her throughout this guide.

The authors have personal experiences with breast cancer. Luanna and her husband Ian experienced many of the diagnostic, surgical, chemotherapy, and reconstruction treatment procedures covered in this book. Steve, alongside his wife Megumi, experienced these as well as other treatment procedures. Luanna, Ian, Steve, and Megumi also encountered many of the side effects associated with breast cancer treatments, the difficult decisions that must be made regarding treatments, and the challenges of staying healthy and communicating about the breast cancer to family and friends.

1 How to Help Someone Thrive with Breast Cancer: An Introduction to This Guide

You are probably reading this Guide because you are a spouse, partner, friend, colleague, or family member of a woman who is experiencing, or is about to experience, the many challenges that accompany breast cancer and its treatments. You want to know how to best support her, what to do and say, and what not to do and say.

Many studies have documented the mental and physical health benefits of support from friends and family during stressful times. Being worried about, or receiving, a diagnosis of breast cancer is a major life stressor that can lead to anxiety, depression, sleep loss, couple distress, disruptions in interactions with friends and family, changes in lifestyle, and many other adverse effects. The treatments for breast cancer and their side effects can also be stressful. Your emotional and practical support could help improve the quality of her life and the likelihood that her cancer treatments will be successful.

The best ways to support a woman with breast cancer depend on many things. First, they depend on your relationship. Maybe you are married or her intimate partner. Perhaps you are a good friend, son or daughter, sister or brother, parent, or work colleague. If you are a friend or family member who can only visit and help sometimes, your role may be less intense but also important. Regardless of your relationship, you can also be affected by her cancer and its treatments.

Women with breast cancer can differ in many ways. They can differ in the type and severity of their breast cancer as well as their age, underlying health and medical history, health insurance and economic resources, and many other personal and social aspects of their lives. They can also differ in their cultural and ethnic background, level of education, number and age of children, relationships with husbands or partners, sexual and gender expression, rural or urban living environment, access to transportation and specialized treatment, work or school responsibilities, and number and type

DOI: 10.4324/9781003194088-1

of friends and family supports. Women with breast cancer can also differ in their physical and emotional reactions to the cancer diagnosis and treatments. These differences affect the best ways to support her.

There are also many aspects of her breast cancer and its treatments with which you could be involved. Perhaps you were with her when she was told of the diagnosis or when she came to a clinic for a biopsy. Perhaps she asked you to help in discussions with her doctor about treatment options. Maybe you accompany her to chemotherapy or radiation sessions. Perhaps you help with injections at home or with her daily living tasks.

It is also possible you are not intimately involved with her daily life or treatment but want to provide emotional and practical support and let her know you care and want to help. Regardless of your relationship and your level of involvement in her treatment, you want to provide meaningful support for her during this challenging time.

The best ways to provide support also depend on her wishes. Research has shown that people differ in their need for support and in the types of support they find most helpful. Some are appreciative of emotional, tangible, and informational support while others may find this demeaning, intrusive, and unhelpful. A recommendation we offer many times in this Guide – offer your support and ask her what would be most helpful. Don't assume that the kinds of support that work for you or for others would also work for her.

Breast Cancer Can Also Affect Supporters

Most people understand that breast cancer can have devastating effects on many aspects of a woman's life. Research has also shown that a woman's breast cancer can affect the people who care about and support her. Breast cancer can have an especially profound effect on persons who are intimately involved in helping someone with its challenging treatment and recovery phases. If you are a spouse, partner, or live together, not only will you be intensely involved with all aspects of her breast cancer and its treatment, they will also affect you.

Regardless of your supporting role, you may also have to cope with your own life disruptions, concerns, and anxieties associated with her cancer and its treatment. If you are her intimate partner, her breast cancer can affect your relationship, how and what the two of you talk about to each other and to friends and family members, how you spend time together, what you eat, your sex life, and your own emotional and physical health. While an important goal of yours is to provide the best emotional and practical support for her, it is crucial that you also maintain your own emotional and physical health. We discuss ways to achieve both of these goals throughout this Guide, especially in Chapter 14.

It is Not Only What to Say and Do, It is Also What Not to Say and Do

It can be difficult to know what to say to a person who is dealing with a life-changing illness like breast cancer. A woman who is usually optimistic, happy, social, energetic, independent, and vigorous can become less so when she is coping with or recovering from breast cancer. She may be tired more often, less optimistic, and less mobile. When you enter the room or call her on the phone, should you say, "How are you feeling?" when you know she is feeling lousy? She may feel grateful if you ask how she is feeling, a sign that you care, or she may think "What a stupid question. Obviously, I feel crappy – I have breast cancer and the drugs are killing me." Should you make some positive comment, "You look rested today?" Or would it be better to avoid any cancer-related topics and talk instead about sports, movies, or family?

Not knowing what to say or being afraid to say the wrong thing can lead to stilted conversations. This discomfort can even lead you, and perhaps some friends and family members, to spend less time with her than you would otherwise. A further complication is that *her preferences for support can change over time.* Chapter 11 offers more ideas about what to say to and about her and how to help others say and do the most helpful things.

The Authors' Backgrounds and Experiences with Breast Cancer

In the following sections, we introduce our experiences with breast cancer. We briefly talk about each of our personal involvements with breast cancer and expand on these in subsequent chapters that discuss the various aspects of breast cancer diagnosis, treatment, and recovery. Two of us, Stephen and Ian, are husbands of women who have experienced breast cancer. Luanna, Ian's wife, is a breast cancer survivor and also provided emotional and practical support for her sister and for a close friend, both with breast cancer.

Stephen's Background and Experience with Breast Cancer

My experience with breast cancer began with a phone call from my wife Megumi's physician while Megumi was visiting her family in Japan.

Megumi and I had arranged for her doctor to inform me about the results of her biopsy. Her biopsy results indicated that she had breast cancer in her left breast – initially diagnosed as a noninvasive form (DCIS) but later upgraded to a more invasive form (IDC) of breast cancer (see Chapter 2 for a description of the types and stages of breast cancer). She had experienced no symptoms, but the biopsy followed two mammograms that had identified suspicious areas. I immediately called Megumi to inform her. I was visiting the Hawaiian island of Maui with my friend Frank when I got the call and, in a sign of my future difficulties in coping with her breast cancer, walked into a restaurant, ordered three margaritas, and walked out forgetting to pay.

That call was my introduction to two years of multiple breast cancer treatments and six additional years of her recovery following the treatments, which still continues. During that time she experienced most of the medical procedures we describe in this Guide – biopsies, two lumpectomies, months of chemotherapy, home injections, fatigue, hair loss, difficulty thinking, hot flashes, weeks of radiation, a mastectomy, reconstructive surgery, and hormone therapy.

That phone call also began my experiences with the many ways her breast cancer and its treatments would affect both of us and the challenges I would face in being a good supporter for her. I believed at the time, incorrectly, that I was handling the personal stress of Megumi's breast cancer superbly. I am a clinical psychologist and know a lot about ways to cope with stress. I have also had to deal with my own physical and health challenges. I later realized I was having difficulties – in talking to others about her breast cancer, maintaining my usual work activities, sleeping well, and avoiding dysfunctional coping strategies, such as alcohol use. My symptoms of distress were sometimes an additional source of stress for her and often she had to reassure me that "everything will be OK."

Some of my adverse effects still occur, more than six years after she started her recovery and is now increasingly healthy and active – she runs several miles a day, is planning to play in an international basketball tournament, is optimistic and happy, her hair has grown back, and she has no signs of cancer from her recent mammograms. Like many cancer survivors, she took hormone medication for years after her treatments to reduce the chance of recurrence or a new cancer. She will also undergo yearly evaluations and consultations with oncology professionals.

My personal stress and not-always-functional reactions and dysfunctional coping responses did not keep me from helping her in many ways. I never missed a cancer doctor's appointment and talked rationally with oncology nurses and doctors (although with insufficient knowledge of breast cancer at the time). I was able to administer injections at home, assisted with home maintenance and daily living tasks, and tried to be emotionally supportive.

When Megumi was diagnosed with breast cancer, I was an Emeritus Professor of psychology at the University of Hawaii. Megumi and I had been married for six years. Up to that time I had only minimal academic knowledge about breast cancer. I was a psychology professor for 40 years and helped develop a quality-of-life measure for cancer patients and struggled through many charity 5-K races for breast cancer without knowing much about the disease for which I was running, ever so slowly, and financially supporting albeit minimally. Importantly, I was especially unaware of the many ways breast cancer would affect her, me, our lives together, and I was unprepared to be the best partner I could be. It has taken me years to learn about this complex disease and its ramifications. Every week while working on this Guide, I had an "I wish I had known this then" experience. One important take-away for me from these experiences is that a healthy and useful strategy to deal with reactions to health problems in someone I care about is to accept them, understand that your reactions are normal, and that you can still be an effective source of support.

Luanna's Background and Experience with Breast Cancer

Breast cancer became personal for me at age 45 when my younger sister of 43 was diagnosed and underwent a lumpectomy. Her treatment was not successful, and the cancer metastasized throughout her body; she died less than two years later at age 45. We lived in different U.S. states, but I traveled to spend time with her and offered my support when I could. Our parents were retired and lived close to her. They had been models of resilience throughout their lives but not in this instance. I don't think they ever recovered emotionally from losing a daughter to cancer; their recurring line was "It is terribly unfair for children to die before their parents." They were so devastated they sold their ideal retirement home and moved across the country to avoid being close to painful memories.

My next personal experience was while we were living in New Zealand. A close colleague and friend of mine was diagnosed with breast cancer, and as she lived alone with no close family nearby, she agreed to allow me to be her support person. I attended doctor's appointments with her in a non-speaking role as note-taker so we could later discuss what was said. She chose a simple mastectomy of the one breast, and I cancelled an international trip to move temporarily into her spare bedroom as support after her operation. I helped her with her drain while she showered, so I saw what a mastectomy looks like and what a drain entails. She chose a prosthesis, not breast reconstruction, and the receptor characteristics of her cancer made it possible to prescribe Tamoxifen to reduce the chance of breast cancer recurrence.

Cancer became harsh reality for me seven years ago, when I was diagnosed with a particularly aggressive form of breast cancer (triple negative invasive ductal carcinoma) of the right breast. I had just had a mammogram six months prior revealing no abnormalities, but a constant sharp, tiny pain in one location in that breast sent me to my doctor. I had never before heard that pain was a symptom for cancer, but I knew something was wrong. Another mammogram was scheduled immediately (again, showing no tumor) followed by another imaging test (magnetic resonance imagery, MRI) that revealed a tiny tumor less than a centimeter in size. My oncologist recommended chemotherapy followed by surgery, and because triple negative tumors are particularly aggressive with lower survival rates, I was scheduled for 12-weeks of chemo almost immediately.

It took a couple of chemo sessions before it happened, but I lost all my hair. It grew back again later, of course, but being bald kept me inside more than I liked because I found wearing a wig (or even a scarf) unbearably hot and uncomfortable.

The surgery was scheduled about a month after the fourth and final chemotherapy session. I recall the oncologist and surgeon advising mastectomy over lumpectomy, but I would have done that anyway as I was determined at that point to get it over with. I also suspected a different choice might have saved my sister's life. I chose a bilateral mastectomy (removal of both breasts) because the tumor was so small it seemed to me there could be even smaller ones already in both breasts. The biopsy of breast tissue during my surgery did reveal a second, even smaller tumor in the right breast but nothing in the left, but I have no regrets about my decision. I agreed prior to surgery that if the testing of three sentinel lymph nodes revealed cancer, all nearby lymph nodes would then also be removed; fortunately, they tested negative. I dreaded the implications of losing lymph nodes under my arm as much as losing my breasts, given possible complications such as permanent fluid build-up in the upper arms. One of my drains was removed a week later, and the drain from my other breast was removed several days after that based on the volume of fluid.

I self-injected an immune booster medication into my belly daily for five days after each of the four chemo sessions. This turned out not to be as bad as it sounds: I found the anticipation of injecting myself worse than the reality of doing it! My chemotherapy included a dose of anti-nausea medication taken by mouth just before chemo injection began at each session. Side effects were minimal, and I never vomited or was even nauseous during chemo.

Because of my family history of cancer (breast cancer in three close women relatives and other cancers in two close male relatives), genetics testing was also advised and covered by my insurance. The 17 genes tested at the time revealed no known cancer-causing mutations, although I was advised to follow up with my genetic counselor every few years and update her on any new personal or family history of cancer. By 2021, over 150 separate genetic mutations associated with cancer had been identified. Hence, a second sequence of genetics testing could reveal a previously unknown hereditary cause for my breast cancer with implications for my blood relatives as well as for my own future cancer screening and prevention.

My health insurance also covered the cost of breast reconstruction; expanders were inserted at the time of the original surgery followed by weekly injections of saline solution. Once the agreed size was reached, another surgery replaced the expanders with silicone implants. Unlike the painful aftermath of the bilateral mastectomy, that final "cosmetic" surgery involved only skin incisions done on an outpatient basis.

In our annual letter to family and friends, my husband and I called that year – after Queen Elizabeth's famous speech – our "annus horribilis." Ian was not only an excellent clinical psychologist, he proved to also be an outstanding support person and husband who took great care of me. After 40+ years as a Professor with expertise in special education, severe disabilities, and educational psychology generally, I was confident I could make decisions that were right for me and fair to Ian and my children. Both of us were experienced researchers and had published extensively in our fields – and even together where our work overlapped – so we knew how to source the scientific literature whenever we had questions or concerns. We respected my doctors, we survived, and there has been no recurrence for the past seven years: I consider myself cured. Triple negative cancers are hormone-resistant, so Tamoxifen or other antiestrogen therapies are not an option for me. Crossing one's fingers and being vigilant are my follow-up regimen! Finally, I need to be honest in revealing that my "breasts" will never be the same and I will always feel that sense of loss. As they say, however, life is far better than the alternative.

Ian's Background and Experience with Breast Cancer

I had never given much thought to cancer other than it being the whispered "Big C" that happened to other people. No one in my immediate family has ever had cancer. I vaguely knew certain cancers were more lethal than others. Media stories of movie stars like Angelina Jolie reporting her double mastectomy seemed especially unfortunate, as though the experience was somehow worse for those who are admired for their physical attributes, even though, as she insisted, not defined by them. My first experience of a patient occurred a long time ago in my private practice after my client read that his cancer could be treated by concentrated mental focus on healthy tissue. As an academic clinical psychologist I had published on the use of mental imagery in psychotherapy. In cancer treatment it is known as *guided imagery*. But as there is no scientific evidence for its effectiveness, I was skeptical. He was adamant, however, I help him as an addition to his medical treatment. I tried introducing such intensive visual imagery as his good cells gobbling up cancer cells like Pac-Man, which had just become popular. After he was admitted to hospice care I visited him for the very last time and he thanked me warmly, though I was greatly saddened that these were his last few days.

In other words, I had only limited notions about cancer – it happened to others, it could be deadly, and breast cancer, which was survivable, meant the loss of attractiveness and positive body image. Nobody would notice if you had missing pancreatic or prostate tissue. Thus I was ill-prepared for my wife's cancer diagnosis, especially as Luanna was always responsible in her self-care – though she'd often grumbled about mammograms being painful and somewhat humiliating.

When the word "chemotherapy" was mentioned in the first big post-diagnosis conference with three doctors present, I cheerfully asked "Soon?" and was taken aback, to put it mildly, when they said "No, tomorrow". It had not dawned on me that the need could be so urgent. I rapidly learned I had to take notes and to ask questions, however basic and naïve they might appear to be. Even then I'd often leave one of these medical consults with only a slim understanding of what was going to happen, what the sequence would be, or what it would mean in practice for Luanna and for us as a couple.

The possibility of her death had never occurred to me until the day of Luanna's mastectomy surgery when I sat in the hospital waiting room much of the day. The surgeon had promised to come out immediately afterwards and tell me how it all went. She did, but about three hours later than she'd predicted. Those were three highly stressful hours.

I hate thinking about unpleasant things, so during that interminable wait I struggled to block my ill-informed mental images of just what exactly the surgeon was doing to Luanna's full and very beautiful breasts. I brooded over the claims of a 4th century Roman historian that Amazon women bound and cut off girls' right breasts so they could be better archers, leaving the left breast intact to feed their babies. My thoughts were rather confused and not very focused on reality. Luanna was less distressed by the chemotherapy than I had expected from the standard assumptions. The surgery, however, required an intensive level of care and accommodations that I performed as best I could, involving mostly small chores and attending to her needs. I did not spend enough time talking with her about what it all meant for our future relationship, other than the practical things, like when she felt ready to drive the car again. I think the stress of the experience made her even more assertive than usual, so much of my strategy was to try to accede to her wishes without making other suggestions and supporting her focus on maintaining her independence. Inevitably, however, I ended up with a lot of time on my hands while she was recuperating, and in those four months wrote my first novel, something I'd been planning in my head since retirement.

I've always recognized the timing of her illness was fortunate, if that word can even be used. I thought it was unfair her first year of her retirement should be taken up with the cancer and that it had led to a cancellation of a major self-guided safari in South Africa, which had taken years of planning. But had her illness appeared earlier it would have more seriously interfered with our move from many years in New Zealand back to Hawai'i, where we both had had our first university jobs. Hawai'i is also medically sophisticated and yet an easy place, climate-wise and socially, in which to manage serious health needs. By this time our children were all older and independent, and with us now being retired, I didn't have to worry about giving up a job to serve as primary support. In all these respects we were extremely privileged.

Lessons Learned

Our personal experiences are consistent with the themes of this Guide: (a) Breast cancer and its treatments can have far-ranging effects on you and her, (b) the more you know about breast cancer, the better able you will be to help both her and you to cope with it, and (c) there are many ways to cope with your stress and the better you can cope with your stress, the better able you and she can thrive in spite of breast cancer.

Complicating anyone's learning about breast cancer is the fact that there is often a lack of consensus among experts on the best methods for detecting and diagnosing breast cancer, the most effective treatments for breast cancer, and the most useful strategies for handling the side effects of treatments. Further, as we are writing this Guide, several major studies have been published or are underway on treatment outcomes; the cost-benefits of mammograms and lumpectomies; new systemic therapies including immunotherapies, targeted therapies, chemotherapies, and hormone therapies; genetic analyses of tumors; and ways to reduce the side effects of chemotherapy. Most of these studies will not affect how you help a woman with breast cancer but if you want to learn more, consult the sources at the end of each chapter and check with her oncology team.

What Is Covered and Not Covered in This Guide?

The goal of this Guide is to suggest ways to help her cope, stay healthy, and thrive as she undergoes this major challenge in her life. A second goal of this Guide is to help you cope, stay healthy, and thrive during this stressful time.

This Guide emphasizes the challenges, difficulties, and opportunities you are likely to encounter in helping a woman with breast cancer. It presents only basic information on the diagnosis, causes, and physiology of breast cancer and breast cancer treatments. However, many sources listed at the end of each chapter present more detailed information on these topics.

This Guide also does not offer treatment recommendations – those are the job of oncology professionals. However, it does discuss the issues she might consider when making treatment decisions in consultation with her oncology team. If you participate with her in making treatment decisions, what questions should be asked? What issues should be considered? If she wishes, you can be emotionally supportive and informative during the decision-making processes but, ultimately, it is important that she makes her treatment decisions in consultation with her oncology team.

We understand as well that people who want to be supportive also differ in many ways. They can differ in their type of relationship and level of intimacy with a woman with breast cancer; availability and job, school, or family obligations; education and health status; reactions to medical procedures; stress-coping skills; and comfort with providing emotional support. This Guide offers many possible ways to provide support during the various phases of breast cancer and its treatment, but the specific ways you choose to be supportive should be decided by you and her. Finally, we suggest ways you can stay healthy during this challenging period of your lives.

Each chapter reviews a particular aspect of breast cancer, outlines the basic issues and procedures, provides recommendations of how you could help, and provides sources for additional information. Chapter 2 presents an overview of the biological basis of breast cancer, its diagnosis and treatments, and the professionals with whom she is likely to meet. Chapter

3 reviews the many decisions that must be made during the diagnosis and treatment of breast cancer and how you can help her decision-making. Chapter 4 discusses how breast cancer is detected, diagnosed, and monitored. Chapters 5–9 discuss common treatments for breast cancer, including lumpectomies and breast-conserving surgery, chemotherapy, radiation, and mastectomies. Chapter 10 deals with breast reconstruction decisions. Chapters 11 and 12 discuss how to talk to family, friends, and children. Chapter 13 concerns later stage cancers with a focus on Stage 4 – cancer that has metastasized beyond the breast – and end-of-life. Chapter 14 focuses on methods to help you cope with stress and keep healthy.

There are many types of cancer other than breast cancer. They differ in their characteristics, causes, effects, progressions, prognosis, treatments, and treatment side effects. Although breast cancer can also occur in men, this Guide is about breast cancer in women.

We recognize that women with breast cancer can more readily receive care if they live in an urban setting with multiple cancer specialists and easy transportation to clinics and hospitals. Many women with breast cancer live in rural areas where cancer specialists and treatment facilities are less accessible. An isolated living situation can present barriers to getting the best diagnostic and treatment options. Presenting additional difficulties, some women with breast cancer are also single mothers, working mothers, or have few nearby family or other social supports.

Although many countries have universal health insurance, the USA does not. Megumi and Luanna had excellent health insurance and financial support through Medicare. Most of the cost of their tests, lumpectomies, surgeries, chemotherapy, radiation treatments, breast reconstruction, and follow-up consultations, were covered by their health insurance and Medicare. The lack of health insurance could have led to delayed detection and treatment. Cost considerations could also affect treatment decisions. We have talked often about how fortunate we were to have good health insurance, easy access to treatment, supportive friends and family, and minimal external obligations. We are aware that many women with breast cancer are much less fortunate.

How This Guide Can Be Used

This Guide is structured so that you can focus on specific chapters that discuss particular aspects of breast cancer, such as how to give her injections at home or some of the possible side effects of chemotherapy. Although each chapter covers specific topics, we recommend you read the entire book because other chapters can provide a useful background and relevant information.

The books, articles, videos, and websites listed at the end of each chapter can help you learn more about specific breast cancer topics. Some websites are only viewable but others provide documents that can be downloaded and printed, usually in PDF format. We have reviewed each source but be warned that, over time, websites change, are updated, become outdated, or are removed. We also provide a detailed subject index at the end of the Guide so that you can easily locate specific topics, such as "lumpectomy," "fatigue," or "hair loss."

We base many recommendations on evidence from well-conducted research studies. Where we have mentioned specific research studies, we include references to the published scientific articles. Some sources are from countries other than the USA or Britain, in order to represent cultural and national differences in the approach to breast cancer.

Where to Learn More about Breast Cancer

We noted that this Guide presents information about breast cancer treatment that was current at the time it was written (2021). However, "best practice" and current knowledge is fluid and has changed even since we started writing. At this moment there are many studies underway on the causes, risk factors, diagnosis, identification and evaluation, prevention, and treatment of breast cancer. As we noted earlier, dozens of public and private agencies in the USA and other countries support breast cancer research and provide research-based information about breast cancer. Some countries have national centers for breast cancer research. To locate these centers, you can do a web search for "breast cancer research funding (name of country)." However, no website we have discovered provides specific and comprehensive guides for ways to support a woman with breast cancer.

There are dozens of well-written and informative guides and websites to help women understand and cope with this disease. Many articles, books, and websites have been written by articulate and insightful women who have survived breast cancer. Others have been written for cancer patients by equally articulate and insightful oncology nurses and physicians and two by husbands of a breast cancer survivor. We have reviewed all of the sources listed in "Sources for More Information" at the end of each chapter and have found them useful. We have attempted to provide the best information and sources of information available at the time we are writing this book.

Our main point here is, if you want more information, check recommended websites for the most recent updates on all of the topics in this book. This is especially important if you are helping her make decisions about surgical, medicine, radiation, and other treatments following a breast cancer diagnosis or a tentative diagnosis.

Useless and sometimes harmful information about breast cancer often appears, especially on the web and in social media. Consider recent titles such as: "Baking Soda Cures Cancer"; "Cancer Cured in 3 Minutes"; "What the Cancer Industry Doesn't Want You to Know"; "Cancer Cure Found!"; "Cancer Cures itself ..."; "Miracle Drug....."

Always consider the source of information and what evidence there is for any recommended treatment. What is the evidence to back-up the claims? Always rely on well-respected organizations that make research-based recommendation. The American Cancer Society, the National Cancer Institute, the Breast Cancer Research Foundation, National Comprehensive Cancer Network, and national cancer centers in other countries are good examples of organizations that promote research on breast cancer and its treatment.

As we mentioned, the cancer specialists we have encountered have been well informed about the results of recent research. However, not all medical professionals may be as well informed and well-informed medical professionals can disagree about diagnoses and treatment recommendations. A second opinion can help allay concerns and increase confidence in treatment decisions. Most specialists will be comfortable with seeking a second opinion. Support her if she is considering asking for a second opinion from other cancer specialists. Perhaps she is afraid of offending her current doctor, and you can reassure her it is normal practice and many people request a second opinion.

Summary and Recommendations

- The best ways to support a woman with breast cancer will depend on her preferences and your relationship with her.
- Your support can help improve the quality of her life and the likelihood that her cancer will be successfully treated.
- There are important differences among women with breast cancer and breast cancer survivors in the best ways to provide support. Each woman who experiences breast cancer is unique in her situation, characteristics, and reactions.
- Let her know that you want to be helpful and ask her what kinds of support would be helpful to her.
- The types of support that works best can change over time.
- An important goal of yours must be to maintain your own emotional and physical health, for your sake and hers.

- The healthiest and most useful strategy to deal with your adverse reactions to breast cancer in someone you care about is to accept them, understand they are normal, and that you can still be an effective support for her despite them.
- Check recommended websites for the most recent updates on all of the topics in this book.
- Always consider the source of information and what evidence there is for any treatment that is being considered; useless and sometimes harmful information about breast cancer often appears.
- Support her if she is considering asking for a second opinion from other cancer specialists.

Sources for More Information

https://www.cancer.net/cancer-types/breast-cancer (the website of the American Society of Clinical Oncology)

https://www.cancer.net/es/tipos-de-cancer/c%C3%A1ncer-de-mama (a website in Spanish)

https://www.cancer.org/cancer/breast-cancer.html (the breast cancer website of the American Cancer Society)

https://www.breastcanceruk.org.uk/ (website in the UK on breast cancer)

https://www.breastcancer.org (a website for information about breast cancer and its treatments)

https://www.canada.ca/en/public-health/services/chronic-diseases/cancer/breast-cancer.html (the website on breast cancer by the Government of Canada)

https://www.bcna.org.au/ (the website of the Breast Cancer Network of Australia)

https://www.cdc.gov/cancer/breast (the website about breast cancer by the Center for Disease Control and Prevention)

https://www.nccn.org/patientresources/patient-resources/guidelines-for-patients (a guide for patients by the National Comprehensive Cancer Network)

https://breast.predict.nhs.uk/ (Predict is a website in the UK that uses data from similar women to predict the likely proportion of such women expected to survive up to 15 years after their surgery with different treatment combinations)

https://www.cdc.gov/spanish/cancer/breast/ (the website in Spanish about breast cancer by the Center for Disease Control and Prevention)

2 Breast Cancer Diagnosis, Treatment, and Providers: An Introduction and Overview

This chapter presents basic information about breast cancer to help you better understand what a woman with breast cancer could experience during diagnosis and treatment. It describes what breast cancer is, how it is detected, and the treatments for breast cancer. The chapter describes the types, structure, and physiology of breast cancer cells; how they are detected and diagnosed; and current science-based treatments of breast cancer. The chapter also identifies the professionals a woman with breast cancer is likely to encounter. Topics introduced in this chapter are discussed in greater detail in subsequent chapters.

This chapter is not a substitute for discussions with oncology specialists or for consulting the more detailed information contained in other chapters and sources. *With a basic understanding of breast cancer and its treatment, you may be better able to offer her support during challenging times.* Recall from Chapter 1 that the information on breast cancer presented in this Guide was current at the time it was written, late 2021. As a supporter, you and she can *consult with her oncology team and the resources listed at the end of each chapter for updated information.*

What Is Breast Cancer?

Breast cancer is the uncontrolled growth of cells in the breast. The genes within a cell usually maintain their orderly replacement and division throughout their life. In breast cancer, changes in genes within a cell in the breast cause it to divide rapidly and uncontrollably, eventually forming a tumor composed of many cancer cells. Some of these cells may travel to other parts of the breast or body and begin to divide and form new tumors.

Not all tumors are dangerous. Some tumors grow slowly and do not spread to other parts of the body or invade nearby tissues. These tumors are considered *benign*. Other tumors are more dangerous because they grow more quickly and can spread to other parts of the body. These

DOI: 10.4324/9781003194088-2

tumors are considered *malignant*. Tumors in the breast that are malignant are labeled as *breast cancer*. Some of the diagnostic procedures discussed in this and other chapters are designed to identify tumors and to see if a tumor is benign or malignant. Treatment decisions are affected by whether a tumor is malignant or benign.

Breast cancer often begins in the milk-producing glands of the breast or the ducts that pass milk from these glands to the nipple. Sometimes, breast cancer can begin in the fatty and fibrous connective tissues of the breast.

Cancer cells are especially dangerous when they spread within the breast and to other parts of the body. One of the first places they can migrate to is the lymph nodes under the arm. These clusters of small organs help maintain the health of a person by filtering out viruses, bacteria, and other foreign substances in the body. A cancer cell that is found in a lymph node is a concern because it indicates that the cancer cells have migrated away from the original tumor in the breast. As we discuss in Chapters 5 and 6, to detect the possible spread of cancer cells, some lymph nodes under the arm may be removed during initial surgeries, such as a lumpectomy, and examined under a microscope.

Types of Breast Cancer

After a suspicious area of a woman's breast has been examined under a microscope (as part of a *biopsy*; see Chapter 5), she will be told by her doctor if the cells are malignant or not. If the cells are malignant, she will also be told the type of the breast cancer. The type of breast cancer is important information because it also affects treatment decisions and the likelihood of successful treatment.

There are many types and subtypes of breast cancer, such as invasive, noninvasive, metastatic, and molecular. The website https://www.breastcancer.org/symptoms/types lists 14 different types and subtypes of breast cancer. A woman with suspected breast cancer will receive a specific diagnosis from her primary doctor or oncologist based on information from a pathologist who examines the cells following the biopsy, which involves the removal of a small part of breast tissue containing the suspected cancer cells. Factors that affect a diagnosis of the type of breast cancer include its location, appearance, and features, whether or not it has migrated to other parts of the breast or body, and its sensitivity to specific hormones (estrogen and progesterone; see Chapter 4 on the diagnosis of breast cancer).

The specific type of breast cancer affects decisions about which treatments might be most effective, in what sequence, and what care

---

Box 2.1   Types of Breast Cancer

- *Ductal carcinoma in situ (DCIS)* starts inside the milk ducts and is noninvasive – the cancer cells haven't spread to other parts of the breast. Although DCIS is not life-threatening and is not considered cancer by some, there is about a 15–30% chance the cancer will transform into an invasive cancer within 10 years. Thus, it is treated aggressively. There is no "lump" or discomfort and most cases of DCIS are first discovered through mammography (see p. 44 below and p. 48 in Chapter 4).
- *Invasive ductal carcinoma (IDC)* is the most common type of invasive breast cancer. In IDC the cancer began in the milk ducts, as in DCIS, but the cancer cells have spread to the surrounding breast tissues. Most often, IDC is discovered through mammography and follow-up biopsies but can also be first noticed through breast pain, swelling of part of the breast, a lump in the breast or underarm, or other changes in the breast. As with DCIS, treatments vary with the characteristics of the cancer and may involve lumpectomy, chemotherapy, lymph node surgery, radiation, mastectomy, and/ or hormonal therapy.
- *Invasive lobular carcinoma (ILC)* is the second most common type of invasive breast cancer. In ILC, the cells have begun to invade the tissues of the breast, often the lymph nodes, and sometimes other areas of the body. ILC is most often initially identified in mammograms with follow-up biopsies. Sometimes, early signs of ILC involve changes in the appearance or sensitivity of the breast and nipple and/or fluid discharge from the nipple.
- *Tubular carcinoma* is a subtype of IDC and is characterized by small tumors composed of tube-like cancer calls. Most often tubular carcinomas are discovered through mammography and biopsies. This cancer is invasive but less so than some others. Prognosis is good because it typically responds well to treatment.

---

might be necessary following successful treatment. It also affects the likelihood of successful treatment and the likelihood that breast cancer will come back after initial successful treatment. Treatments vary with the type and characteristics of the cancer and may involve lumpectomy, radiation, mastectomy, chemotherapy, and/or hormonal therapy, which are discussed below and in subsequent chapters.

A few common types of breast cancer are listed in Box 2.1 but her doctor will provide a more specific diagnosis and discuss its implications for treatment. Types of breast cancer are also described in https://www.nationalbreastcancer.org/types-of-breast-cancer.

Stages of Breast Cancer

If cancer cells are identified during a biopsy of breast tissue or lymph nodes, she will be given information about the *stage* of the breast cancer. In the USA, the stage of breast cancer gives an estimate of how advanced the cancer is according to how large it is, its appearance and features, and whether it has spread to other parts of the breast or other parts of the body. The stage of cancer also reflects whether or not it is producing specific proteins and is sensitive or resistant to estrogen and progesterone. The information from a biopsy may be augmented with information from physical exams, or PET/CT scans, bone scans, and blood tests where advanced cancer is suspected.

In the UK, a similar system is referred to as TNM — Tumor size, the number of positive Nodes, and absence/presence of Metastases (the spread of cancer cells to areas outside the breast). Each letter is accompanied by a number that corresponds to severity. However, most oncologists in the UK categorize a cancer as either *Primary* (equivalent to Stages I-III) or *Secondary* (equivalent to Stage IV or advanced cancer; see Box 2.2).

In the American system, there are five stages of breast cancer (0–IV, see Box 2.2), although only four of these – Stages I–IV – are generally regarded as cancer. Information about breast cancer can also be communicated in terms of location and spread:

> *Local*: The cancer has not been found outside of the breast.
> *Regional*: The cancer has been found also in the lymph nodes.
> *Distant*: The cancer is also found also in other parts of the body.

The higher stages represent the severity and degree of spread of cancer; they are associated with higher health risks and decreasing survival rates. Stages of breast cancer and their treatment options are also discussed in https://www.breastcancer.org/symptoms/types and in several other websites listed at the end of this chapter.

Box 2.2   Stages of Breast Cancer

- *Stage 0*: Stage 0 describes breast cancer that is noninvasive – it started in the milk ducts and glands and has not invaded nearby tissue. DCIS (ductal carcinoma in situ) is a common form of Stage 0. Some oncologists don't consider DCIS as true breast cancer.
- *Stage I:* Stage I describes breast cancer that has invaded nearby tissue. Stage I is divided into subcategories IA and IB, depending on the size, location, hormone sensitivity, and whether or not it has reached the lymph nodes.
- *Stage II*: Stage II also describes breast cancer that has invaded nearby tissue. Stage II is divided into subcategories IIA and IIB depending on the size, location, hormone sensitivity, and whether or not it has reached beyond the first or second lymph node.
- *Stage III*: Stage III breast cancer tends to be larger, more invasive, and has migrated to more lymph nodes compared to Stages I and II.
- *Stage IV*: Stage IV describes breast cancer that is more invasive than that of previous stages and is often called Metastatic Breast Cancer or Secondary Breast Cancer (see Chapter 13). In this stage, cancer cells have migrated to other organs of the body such as the liver, lungs, bones, and brain.

Hormone Receptor Status of Cancer Cells

Cancer cells differ in their genetic make-up and these differences affect how they respond to a woman's hormones (estrogen and progesterone). A cancer cell's hormone sensitivity affects which medicines might be most effective in treating the cancer. Box 2.3 and https://www.breastcancer.org/symptoms/types/molecular-subtypes describe genetic/molecular subtypes of breast cancer.

Risk Factors for Breast Cancer

Research has identified many factors associated with the risk that a woman will develop breast cancer. Many of these factors cannot be controlled. Factors that increase the risk of breast cancer include age,

Box 2.3   Types of Breast Cancer Based on Their Genetics and Hormone Sensitivity

- *Estrogen receptor positive (ER+)*: Estrogen promotes the growth of the cancer cells.
- *Progesterone receptor positive (PR+)*: Progesterone promotes the growth of the cancer cells.
- *Hormone receptor negative (HR-)*: The cancer cells are not affected by hormones and hormone-blocking medicines will not be effective.
- *HER2 status*: The HER2 tests indicate if the HER2 gene is affecting the growth of the cancer cells (HER2+ = positive or HER2- = negative). Specific medicines can be prescribed if the cancer cells are identified as HER2 positive. Detailed information about HER2, tests for HER2, and medicines prescribed for HER2 positive cancers can be found at https://www.breastcancer.org/symptoms/diagnosis/her2.
- *Triple-negative*: The cancer cells are ER-, PR-, and HER2-. The cancer cells are not affected by hormone therapy medicines or medicines that target HER2 receptors. They tend to grow faster than other cancers and have a poorer prognosis. The cancer is often treated with chemotherapy followed by surgery. Women with triple-negative breast cancer are advised to cease taking any hormone dosage previously prescribed to mitigate menopausal symptoms and are treated with neoadjuvant chemotherapy (see Chapter 7).
- *HER2-enriched*: The cancer cells are ER-, PR-, and HER+ HER2-enriched cancers tend to grow faster than luminal cancers and have a worse prognosis. Specific medicines can be prescribed if the cancer cells are identified as HER2 positive.

female sex (many more women than men develop breast cancer), a family history of breast cancer, genetic factors, a history of abnormal breast cells, early menstruation, and dense breast tissue. Research has also identified additional personal factors that can increase the risk of breast cancer. These include physical inactivity, poor diet, being overweight, alcohol and tobacco use, pregnancy and breast-feeding history, and hormone replacement therapy. The risk of breast cancer is also slightly higher for some ethnic minority groups. Research has also suggested that the risk of breast cancer is likely associated with exposure to some environmental factors, such as pesticides, some man-made chemicals, toxins, and pollutants.

An important point for the caregiver is that, in most cases, it is unlikely that the cause of a particular woman's breast cancer can be known. Another important point is that 60–70% of breast cancer patients had no known risk factors. She and others may wonder if she did something wrong that caused her breast cancer – *you can reassure her, and others, that she is not responsible for her breast cancer.*

Many myths and disinformation about the causes of breast cancer are spread through social media. We know the risk of breast cancer *is not* associated with cell phones, microwaves, contact with breast cancer patients, particular clothing, mammograms, the use of deodorants, implants, bras, having an abortion or miscarriage, and hair dye. For more information on the risks for breast cancer see https://www.nationalbreastcancer.org/breast-cancer-risk-factors and https://www.cdc.gov/cancer/breast/basic_info/risk_factors.htm.

How You Can Help

As a caregiver, you can promote one of this Guide's key directives: *Every woman should talk to her oncology team about her type and stage of cancer and continue these discussions until she understands the implications for her health and treatment options.* We discuss in Chapter 3 the many ways you can help her in these discussions.

Information about the type and stage of breast cancer is a lot to take in and, understandably, some of it may be stressful for her (and you) to hear. Being told the cancer is advanced or particularly aggressive can be particularly worrying. We know from lots of research that when people are under stress, they have more difficulty taking in information and making good decisions. *So, offer to go with her so you can be an extra set of ears and take notes during these important consultations.* With the doctor's permission you may be able to record the discussion for later review.

How Breast Cancer Is Detected, Diagnosed, and Monitored

Several methods are used to detect, diagnose, and monitor breast cancer and its treatment effects. Mammogram, magnetic resonance imagery (MRI), ultrasound, biopsies, and blood tests are the most often used. These procedures, and suggestions for how you can help her prepare for them, are discussed in greater detail in Chapters 4–5. Other methods are currently being investigated and her doctor will explain them if they are being considered.

Mammogram and 3D Mammogram

As we discuss in Chapter 4 (p. 44), a mammogram is an X-ray of the breast that allows a specialist to identify any suspicious areas. If it is a regular mammogram for a woman without breast cancer symptoms it is called a *screening mammogram*. If it is a mammogram for a woman who has breast cancer symptoms or indictors, it is called a *diagnostic mammogram*. Mammograms can't diagnose cancer, but they can indicate if additional tests are needed to help with a diagnosis.

A *three-dimensional mammograms* (i.e., 3D mammogram or *breast tomosynthesis*) is sometimes recommended for younger women or women with dense breast tissue. During a 3D mammogram, each breast is compressed once and X-rays are taken from different angles. The images are then combined in a computer for a three-dimensional view of the breast.

The radiologist who examines her mammogram will give their impressions to her doctor. The American College of Radiology has established the BI-RADS as a uniform way to describe the results of mammogram imaging and their implications for follow-up. These are described in Box 4.1 (p. 48).

Magnetic Resonance Imagery (MRI)

Breast MRI uses radio waves and magnets with specially designed equipment to make pictures of the inside of the breast. MRI is often used with women who have been diagnosed with breast cancer in order to precisely locate tumors in the breast and measure their size.

The MRI scan can take an hour or more while she is inside a tube-like enclosure. During that time, the woman must remain immobile and avoid movements that would interfere with the results. Some patients may feel anxious inside the enclosure and she will be able to temporarily stop the test if she becomes distressed.

Chapter 4 (p. 47) describes the MRI procedure in greater detail and Box 4.3 (p. 50–51) discusses ways you can help her prepare for and cope if she is feeling anxious before or during the MRI. She can also request medication to help her relax.

Biopsies

If a mammogram identifies possible cancer cells, a *biopsy* will be performed to find out if the cells are benign or malignant. There are several types of biopsies (see Box 5.1 in Chapter 5) but all involve the removal and examination under a microscope of a section of the suspicious tissue or fluid from the breast. Most biopsies are performed with local anesthesia and sometimes with a light general anesthesia or medications to help the woman relax during the procedure. The tissue samples taken during a biopsy are sent to a pathologist for examination. The pathologist will send their report to the patient's oncology doctor after the tissue is examined (See Chapter 5 for more information on biopsies).

Ultrasound

In an *ultrasound* examination, sound waves are used to make computer pictures of the inside of the breast. It is often used to examine lumps and cysts in the breast, to guide the needle used in biopsies, and as a follow-up to mammograms. It can be especially useful with women who have dense breasts. During the procedure, the breast is covered with a thin gel and a wand which emits high-frequency sound waves (which cannot be heard) is moved over the breast. The sound waves bounce off breast tissue and the information is transmitted to a computer that produces an image of the breast. When breast cancer has been treated with chemotherapy or radiation, an ultrasound may also be performed to check for damage to the heart or lungs. See Chapter 4 (p. 51) for more information on ultrasound.

Electrocardiogram and Echocardiogram

Some treatments for breast cancer, such as chemotherapy or whole breast radiation, can affect the heart and lungs. An *electrocardiogram, echocardiogram,* and other heart tests are sometimes performed in a doctor's office or at a hospital to examine the heart muscle, valves, or rhythm for problems before, during, or after cancer treatments.

The tests last about five minutes to one hour, depending on whether it is an electrocardiogram or echocardiogram. First, a woman will lie on her back or side. For the electrocardiogram, wires will then be placed over the heart and during an echocardiogram a wand will be moved over the heart, as described in Chapter 4 (p. 52).

Blood Tests

Breast cancer and chemotherapy can affect many parts of the body and *blood tests* are often used to monitor a woman's overall health, especially the effects of chemotherapy. Blood tests can provide information about the number of white and red blood cells, platelets, proteins, and enzymes. This information is used to guide the schedule and type of chemotherapy that a woman experiences. For example, the schedule of chemotherapy sessions might be changed if a blood test indicates possible liver or kidney damage (see p. 53 in Chapter 4 for more information on blood tests).

Genetic Testing

Because breast cancer is associated with changes in the genes of cells, some women with breast cancer may be referred for genetic testing and counseling. According to the American Cancer Society, about 5–10% of breast cancers are thought to result from inherited mutations in specific genes. These tests can be helpful in indicating if close relatives, such as daughters, sisters, granddaughters, or mothers, have an elevated risk for cancer. They can also indicate if there are mutations in the *BRCA1* and *BRCA2* genes. Because of the close link between these genes and breast cancer, women with one of these gene changes (called Hereditary Breast and Ovarian Cancer Syndrome) sometimes choose to have a preventive mastectomy to reduce the chance of cancer recurrence or of cancer in the other breast, even when no cancer cells have been found.

Genetic testing can involve cells that are not cancerous (germline/hereditary genetic testing) or cells with somatic gene mutations (genetic mutations acquired during the formation of cancer cells). A genetic counselor will develop a family history of cancer and arrange for genetic testing. A referral for genetic counseling and testing is more likely if the woman is younger; has a family history of breast cancer; triple-negative breast cancer, been diagnosed with other cancers or breast cancer a second time; or be of Ashkenazi Jewish descent. The test involves sending a sample of blood or saliva to a laboratory for testing. The indications for genetic testing and the genes that are tested are constantly evolving. Hereditary factors in breast cancer are discussed in: https://www.cdc.gov/genomics/disease/breast_ovarian_cancer/index.htm

For more information on genetic testing, see https://www.cancer.org/cancer/breast-cancer/risk-and-prevention/genetic-testing.html

How You Can Help During Detection, Diagnosis, and Monitoring

In subsequent chapters we discuss many ways you can help her before, during, and after testing and diagnostic procedures. Some of these tests, and receiving information about the results of the tests, can be stressful. It can be difficult to think clearly when under stress. Our main recommendation – *Be an informed supporter.* You will be better able to help her if you are informed about the procedures and potential results of the tests. As we recommend in Chapters 1 and 3, *if she wishes, help her talk with her oncology team about the procedures and their implications, understand the information the doctor is giving her, and make good treatment decisions. If she agrees, accompany her to the clinic, provide transportation, discuss the procedures, take notes, and provide comfort and support afterward. When she receives the results, you will be in a better position to help her clarify their implications with the oncologist.*

Breast Cancer Treatments

There are many treatment options for breast cancer. They differ in how invasive they are and in their side effects. Each type of treatment can vary in its duration, severity, and specific aspects, depending on the type and stage of her cancer, her medical history and health, her experience with previous treatments, age, pregnancy status, and preferences. A woman with breast cancer, in consultation with her doctor, should consider the potential benefits, risks, side effects, and possible long-term implications associated with each treatment. Several of the most common treatments are discussed below, and Chapters 6–9 provide more information on specific treatments.

Surgery

Surgery to remove suspected cancer cells is a common treatment for breast cancer. There are several types of surgery (see Box 2.4 and Chapters 6, 9, and 10). Surgery can be used to remove the cancer and to see if the cancer has spread to the lymph nodes or other parts of the breast. Two of the most common surgeries are lumpectomy and mastectomy. A lumpectomy (see Chapter 6) is often performed with a local anesthetic but sometimes with a general anesthetic. Mastectomies (see Chapter 9) are performed under general anesthesia. Reconstructive surgery (Chapter 10) can be used to return the breast to a more normal shape after the cancer has been removed with a lumpectomy or mastectomy.

Box 2.4   Types of Breast Cancer Surgery

• *Lumpectomy* (also called *quadrantectomy, partial mastectomy, or segmental mastectomy*) involves the removal of the part of the breast containing the cancer and some of the surrounding tissue. This surgery allows a woman to keep most of her breast and is often followed by radiation treatment.
• *Mastectomy* involves the removal of the entire breast. Some women without signs of cancer but with particular gene mutations or a strong family history of breast cancer choose *prophylactic mastectomy* which removes one or both breasts to reduce her risk of developing cancer.
• *Partial mastectomy* involves the removal of the part of the breast tissue containing the cancer and some normal tissue around it. Unlike a lumpectomy that removes the cancerous tissue and a small part of the surrounding tissue, a partial mastectomy removes a larger part of the surrounding tissue.
• *Lymph node surgery* involves the surgical removal of lymph nodes, usually those under the arm. *Sentinel lymph node biopsy* involves removal of one or a few lymph nodes under the arm. Its main purpose is to see if the cancer has spread. *Axillary lymph node dissection* involves the removal of many lymph nodes under the arm.
• *Advanced breast cancer surgery* involves removal of cancer cells that have migrated to other parts of the body.

Chemotherapy

Most breast cancer patients receive some form of chemotherapy, either before or after surgery (see Chapter 7). Chemotherapy can be used in early and later stages of breast cancer. It can also be used to attack cancer cells that might have been missed in surgery or that have spread to other parts of the breast and body, to reduce the chance of recurrence of cancer, to shrink a tumor prior to surgery, or to reduce symptoms in advanced cases of breast cancer.

In chemotherapy, drugs are injected into a vein or taken by mouth to kill the cancer cells or to stop them from dividing. Chemotherapy injections often occur in specialized chemotherapy rooms in a hospital or clinic but can also occur in a doctor's office or at home. Because some of the chemotherapy medicines are harsh, many women will have a *port* surgically inserted to reduce damage to their veins (see p. 82 in Chapter 7). The frequency, duration, and schedule of chemotherapy sessions depends on the type of cancer, type of medicine used, a woman's health, and how she reacts to the medicine. Some women experience adverse side effects from the chemotherapy drugs (see p. 93, Chapter 7 on side effects of chemotherapy). Chemotherapy drugs work by attacking fast growing or fast replicating cancer cells, but other cells in the body are also fast growing (such as hair and cells in the intestinal track) and the drugs can also attack them. These systemic effects of chemotherapy account for some of its side effects.

Radiation Therapy

Radiation treatments focus high-energy beams on specific areas in the breast, other areas where cancer cells have been detected (such as lymph nodes), or areas where cancer cells have been surgically removed. It is often given several weeks after surgery or chemotherapy to kill any cancer cells that were missed and to reduce the chance the cancer will come back. Radiation for breast cancer can be delivered externally by a large machine or by placing radioactive cancer-killing seeds into the affected area.

Radiation affects all cells that are in the path of the beam, but it affects cancerous cells more. Sessions are painless and side effects associated with external radiation can include fatigue, skin irritation, bruising, and redness at the radiation site. See Chapter 8 for more information on radiation therapy.

Hormone Therapy

Many breast cancer cells (about 80–85%) are sensitive to hormones such as estrogen or progesterone and specific proteins that can stimulate their growth. If tests reveal that a woman's cancer cells are sensitive to estrogen and/or progesterone, hormone therapy after surgery may be recommended. Hormone therapies are intended to slow or stop the growth of cancer cells, to reduce the risk of cancer coming back, or to reduce the risk of new cancers developing. If her cancer cells are hormone-resistant, hormone therapy will not be prescribed and she may even have to cease taking any hormonal medication previously prescribed, such as those to manage post-menopausal symptoms.

There are several possible schedules for hormone therapy and the oncologist will explain the options. A common strategy is for a woman to take specific pills daily, depending on her menopausal status, for 10 years.

The potential side effects of hormone therapy depend on the specific medicine that is taken. Common side effects include hot flashes, night sweats, and vaginal dryness. Less common side effects include blood clots, bone loss, and mood swings, among others.

Chapter 7 provides additional information about hormone therapy.

How You Can Help During Treatments

Subsequent chapters of this Guide offer many practical and socially supportive ways that you could help her prepare for, cope with, and thrive during breast cancer treatments and their side effects. Some of the treatments and their side effects can be uncomfortable and distressing. *Let her know that you would like to help and ask her what would be most helpful.*

Medical Care Providers

Breast cancer is a complex disease and she may have contact with many professionals during detection, diagnosis, treatment, and care. A range of cancer-related health care professionals are described in: https://www.cancer.org/treatment/finding-and-paying-for-treatment/choosing-your-treatment-team/health-professionals-associated-with-cancer-care.html. In addition to a breast cancer patient's primary care provider, she may encounter several of the professionals that are listed below and in Boxes 2.5 and 2.6. A *Medical Oncologist* often coordinates a woman's overall breast cancer treatment. A medical oncologist is a physician with special training in the diagnosis and treatment of cancer who explains, administers, and coordinates the testing, diagnosis, treatment, and post-treatment care. An oncologist usually works with surgeons, nurses, social workers, pathologists, and a woman's primary care provider.

The range of professionals that she is most likely to encounter is listed in Boxes 2.5 and 2.6. Further details on cancer-related health care professionals are also described in: https://www.cancer.org/treatment/finding-and-paying-for-treatment/choosing-your-treatment-team/health-professionals-associated-with-cancer-care.html

Her Treatment Summary and Survivorship Care Plan

At some point during her treatment for breast cancer, her health care provider and oncology team may complete an *Oncology Treatment Summary and Survivorship Care Plan*. The development of these plans was

Box 2.5 Types of Oncology Specialist Often Involved in Breast Cancer Treatment

- *Medical oncologist:* A medical oncologist is a doctor who specializes in the treatment of cancer using chemotherapy or other medications.
- *Surgical oncologist:* A surgical oncologist is a doctor who performs biopsies, lumpectomies, and mastectomies (see Chapters 7–10).
- *Radiation oncologist:* A radiation oncologist is a doctor who treats cancer with radiation and works with radiation therapists and technologists (who administer the radiation treatment), radiation therapy nurses, physicists, and dosimetrists (who plan the correct dose, focus, and rate of radiation therapy) for cancer treatment. A radiation oncologist can also help coordinate post-treatment care (see Chapter 8).
- *Reconstructive/plastic surgeon:* In breast cancer, a reconstructive or plastic surgeon is a doctor who specializes in rebuilding or replacing breast tissue that has been removed during surgery. The surgeon often uses some special material with the right consistency to hold the shape or form of the breast over time (see Chapter 10).
- *Anesthesiologist:* An anesthesiologist is a doctor who specializes in giving medicines that minimize pain, prepare a patient for surgery, or put a patient to sleep before and during surgery, and monitors the patient's recovery after surgery. An anesthesiologist may work with Certified Registered Nurse Anesthetists or Anesthesia Assistants.
- *Pathologist:* A pathologist is a doctor who examines tissues from breast biopsies and surgical samples under a microscope to determine if it's cancer. If it is cancer, the pathologist will also identify the type and grade of the tumor, its genetic characteristics, and its hormone receptor status (see Chapter 5). This information helps the oncologist decide on the best treatment. https://www.mskcc.org/news/what-does-breast-cancer-pathologist-do-work-hannah-wen discusses the role of a pathologist.
- *Physician assistant (PA):* A physician's assistant has a master's or doctoral level degree and is licensed to work collaboratively with, or independently from, a physician, depending on state requirements. Depending on location and applicable regulations,

they may perform examinations, prescribe medications, and administer some treatments.

- *Oncology social worker:* An oncology social worker assists the patient and family on issues such as insurance, education, social support and interactions with friends and family, emotional and spiritual impacts of cancer, stress management, living wills and medical directives, cultural issues in treatment or side effects, psychological and behavioral health, and decision-making.
- *Genetic counselor.* A genetic counselor is a specially trained health professional who discusses with patients the risk of a genetic disorder associated with their breast cancer based on family history and if genetic testing may be helpful. They also discuss the results of genetic testing and some options based on those results, such as recommendations for testing family members.
- *Occupational therapist (OT):* An OT is a specially trained therapist who helps a breast cancer patient overcome functional limitations in daily living and working and helps her to maintain good health following treatment.
- *Physical therapist (PT):* A physical therapist is a specially trained therapist who assists in recovery from some of the effects of lumpectomies, radiation treatments, mastectomies, and breast reconstruction.

initiated in 2014 by the American Society of Clinical Oncology (ASCO) to summarize relevant information about her cancer diagnostic and treatment history. The care plan also recommends follow-up care in the years to come and incorporates both medical advice regarding ongoing monitoring and healthy lifestyle choices to reduce the chance that her cancer will recur. A copy of a 49-page booklet and forms that can be filled out and edited can be found at https://www.cancer.net/survivorship/follow-care-after-cancer-treatment/asco-cancer-treatment-and-survivorship-care-plans.

The oncology treatment summary section includes (a) the names and roles of her oncology team; (b) a family risk assessment including cancer diagnoses in other close family members and any genetic testing results; (c) the details of her breast cancer including the date, type, and the stage of her cancer at initial diagnosis; and (d) cancer treatments and dates for surgeries, radiation, chemotherapy (with lists of specific drugs and dosages), and/or ongoing hormone medications if relevant.

The follow-up care plan includes recommendations to monitor for symptoms of a possible recurrence or other complications, a schedule of

---

Box 2.6   Types of Nurses Involved in Breast Cancer Treatment

- *Registered nurse (RN)*: An RN is a professional nurse registered with the state who has completed a college program in nursing and passed a national examination. RNs are involved in the assessment and treatment of patients throughout the diagnosis, treatment, and follow-up phases of breast cancer. Many attain additional training to become a clinical nurse specialist, nurse practitioner, or nurse anesthetist.
- *Oncology nurse* (sometimes called a *hematology/oncology nurse*): An oncology nurse is an RN with special training in the care of cancer patients and their families. Some nurses receive special training in the administration of chemotherapy drugs.
- *Clinical nurse specialist*: A clinical nurse specialist is an RN with advanced degrees and special training who works closely with the cancer team and may be involved in patient and family care during and after treatment.
- *Licensed practical nurse (LPN)*: An LPN assists registered nurses and physicians and helps with the administration of medicines, monitoring a patient's health status and overall care of a patient.
- *Nurse practitioner*: A nurse practitioner is an RN who has obtained additional training in diagnosis and treatment. Nurse practitioners can prescribe medications and can work collaboratively with, or independently from, physicians, depending on their location and applicable state regulations.
- *Radiation therapy nurse*: A radiation therapy nurse is an RN with advanced training in radiation therapy and the management of its side effects.
- *Nurse anesthetist*: A nurse anesthetist screens patients prior to surgery, administers anesthesia for surgery or other medical procedures, and monitors the patient during anesthesia.

---

clinical visits with the different members of her oncology team, a schedule for future tests and diagnostics, possible long-term side effects from her cancer treatment, resources for more information such as major cancer organization website addresses, and recommendations for healthy post-cancer lifestyle choices.

While most of her treatment summary and survivorship care plan will be specific to her, the lifestyle choice recommendations are likely to be generic. If she wishes, you can discuss with her how to maintain a healthy diet, establish a schedule of regular exercise, get vaccinations, and reduce risk factors such as smoking and alcohol use. If you are her intimate partner, her mother, adult children, or close friends *sharing a healthy lifestyle plan with her can be one of the most important things you can do to help her stay healthy.*

Summary and Recommendations

- An oncology nurse, physician, or other providers and the resources listed at the end of this Guide are good sources for updated information about breast cancer and its treatments.

- Breast cancer is the uncontrolled growth of cells in the breast that can form malignant tumors.

- There are many types, subtypes, stages, and characteristics of breast cancer, which influence decisions about which treatments might be most effective.

- Many controllable and uncontrollable factors affect the risk of developing breast cancer, but 60–70% of breast cancer patients had no risk factors.

- Mammograms, MRIs, ultrasound, biopsies, and blood tests are often used to detect, diagnose, and monitor breast cancer and its treatment effects.

- Genetics testing and counseling is likely to become part of the diagnostic process where there is a strong family history of cancer and/or for particular cancer diagnoses.

- A mammogram is an X-ray used to identify suspicious areas in the breast. Mammograms can be considered screening or diagnostic; 3D mammograms are sometimes recommended for younger women or women with dense breast tissue.

- Breast MRI uses radio waves and magnets with specially designed equipment to make pictures of the inside of the breast, often to locate and measure tumors.

- There are several types of biopsies, but all are performed to see if abnormal cells identified in a mammogram are benign or malignant.

- In an *ultrasound* examination, sound waves are used to make computer pictures of the inside of the breast, to look at abnormal areas in the breast, to guide biopsies, and to see how well blood is flowing inside the breast.

- An ultrasound, electrocardiogram, and/or echocardiogram are used to examine the heart for problems before, during, or after cancer treatments.
- Blood tests are used to provide information about the number of white and red blood cells, platelets, proteins, and enzymes, particularly during chemotherapy.
- Surgery, including lumpectomy, mastectomy, lymph node surgery, and reconstructive surgery are used to remove suspected cancer cells or to return the breast to its presurgical form.
- Chemotherapy can be used in early and later stages of breast cancer as well as in combination with other treatments. It is intended to kill the cancer cells or to stop them from dividing. It affects the whole body through the patient's bloodstream.
- Radiation treatments may be given several weeks after surgery to kill any remaining cancer cells.
- Hormone therapies are intended to reduce the production of hormones or to reduce the ability of hormones to stimulate the growth of cancer cells but will not be relevant to treatment of hormone-resistant cancers.
- A woman undergoing testing or treatment for breast cancer is likely to encounter many medical specialists.
- If she agrees, you can help accompany her to the clinic, provide transportation, discuss the procedures with her, assist in asking the doctor good questions, provide comfort after visits to the doctor and when she receives the results of diagnostic procedures, provide practical help at home, and help clarify their implications with the oncologist.
- Her oncology team may provide her with an oncology treatment summary so that she will have a permanent record of her cancer diagnosis and treatment.
- Support her in the development of her survivorship care plan specific to her circumstances and needs, including information about future monitoring, tests, and procedures.

Sources for More Information

https://www.cancer.net/cancer-types/breast-cancer (the website of the American Society of Clinical Oncology)

https://www.cancer.org/cancer/breast-cancer.html (the breast cancer website of the American Cancer Society)

https://www.breastcanceruk.org.uk/ (website in the UK on breast cancer) https://www.breastcancer.org (a website for information about breast cancer and its treatments)

https://www.canada.ca/en/public-health/services/publications/diseases-conditions/breast-cancer.html# (the website on breast cancer by the Government of Canada)

https://www.bcna.org.au/ (the website of the Breast Cancer Network of Australia)

https://www.cdc.gov/cancer/breast (the website about breast cancer by the Center for Disease Control and Prevention)

https://www.cdc.gov/spanish/cancer/breast/ (the website in Spanish about breast cancer by the Center for Disease Control and Prevention)

https://www.cancer.net/survivorship/follow-care-aftercancer-treatment/asco-cancer-treatment-and-survivorship-care-plans (the ASCO website to obtain a copy of their Treatment Summary and Survivorship Care Plan)

Choi, Y., Smith, K. C., Shukla, A., Blackford, A. L., Wolff, A. C., Thorner, E., Peairs, K. S., ... Synder, C. F. (2020). Breast cancer survivorship care plans: What are they covering and how well do they align with national guidelines? Breast Cancer Research and Treatment, 179, 415–424. Doi: 10.1007/s10549-019-05480-w

3   Helping Her Make Testing and Treatment Decisions

A woman undergoing testing or treatment for breast cancer must make many decisions. For example, if a biopsy identifies cancer cells in the tissue sample, she may have to choose between a lumpectomy and mastectomy. Later, she may have to decide how to cope with adverse effects of chemotherapy and whether or not to have reconstructive surgery. She may also have to decide how to communicate with children, family, and friends about her breast cancer, and how to cope if the treatments for breast cancer were unsuccessful.

Decisions regarding medical care and treatment have serious outcomes and can be complex and stressful. Receiving information that she has breast cancer, or experiencing some of the treatments for breast cancer, can be particularly stressful. Research has shown that when a person is under stress, it can be more difficult for them to absorb and consider information and make the best decisions based on that information. We emphasize in this chapter that your support and help while her doctor is explaining test results and their implications, and your discussions with her about treatment options, could help her make good decisions about her care and treatment.

Decisions Can Be Difficult to Make

Having to make decisions is a feature of everyday life. You've been offered a job in another state, do you really want to move right now? These kinds of choices always have pros (likely advantages) and cons (likely disadvantages). Even deciding between two equally desirable options can be difficult – just watch a young child in an ice cream parlor trying to decide between chocolate chip and caramel crunch!

Psychologists have been studying how people make decisions, how to make the best ones, and errors that people sometimes make in their decision-making. It would be comforting to think that we all carefully

DOI: 10.4324/9781003194088-3

consider the pros and cons of various options and then make the most sensible decisions with the best outcomes. Alas, often, we do not. Sometimes our decisions are influenced by things we remember from past experiences that may not be applicable to the current situation, by what is easiest to understand, by talking with people whose opinions we value, and by information from news reports and social media. Our decisions can also be influenced by what we believe is right or moral, what our friends or neighbors will think of us, or what will be best for others.

Decision-making is particularly stressful for some people. They worry about whether they are making the right decision and to reduce this stress, they may avoid making decisions or make quick decisions without carefully thinking through the options. Our main points here – sometimes, our decisions are based on factors other than what might be best for us!

Research studies have identified factors critical to good decision-making. Some of the most important are access to relevant information and trust in the sources of the information. Even with good information and sources, people differ in the degree to which they are willing to take risks and how much they are influenced by the outcome of their recent decision-making experiences.

Remember that many of the decisions she needs to make can also be influenced by factors other than medical issues and the characteristics of the cancer. Decisions about having a lumpectomy or mastectomy, for example, can be influenced by the degree to which the appearance of her breast is important to her and her concerns about disfigurement. She may also be anxious about the chance the breast cancer will return or new cancers will develop. Many women today are beginning their families at an older age than in previous generations, which puts them in an age range where breast cancer occurs more frequently. This means there will be more cases where someone diagnosed with breast cancer is considering or even planning to have a child or more children in the future. She may opt against treatments for early-stage cancer that can result in early menopause – ruling out pregnancy – or reduce the ability to breastfeed a baby. She may also be unsure if and how to talk to her children, family, and friends about her breast cancer.

This chapter briefly reviews some of the decisions that she may need to make during the course of her breast cancer diagnosis and treatment. All are considered in greater depth in other chapters. Next, this chapter presents strategies to help you help her with decision-making and offers suggestions about how to talk with her when she is making diagnostic or treatment decisions about her breast cancer. We emphasize your role as a supporter – always, the decisions are hers to make.

Box 3.1   Decision-Making During Diagnosis and Treatment

- Even before a diagnosis, a younger woman will have to decide whether or not to have a screening mammogram (see Chapter 4, p. 45).
- Should she seek a second opinion about the results of a biopsy (see Chapter 1, p. 13 and Chapter 4, p. 66)?
- She may be offered the opportunity to participate in a research study comparing different treatments. These are usually in the form of a "randomized controlled trial" that involves groups of volunteer patients who are randomly selected to receive the new treatment, the usual treatment, or a placebo (a harmless substance). Her doctor will explain what her participation would involve and the benefits and risks of participating.
- Should she have another biopsy, a lumpectomy, or a mastectomy following a positive finding from the first biopsy (see Chapter 6, p. 68; Chapter 9, p. 124)?
- If cancer cells were identified at the margins of the tissue sample after a second lumpectomy, should she choose a third lumpectomy, a partial mastectomy, or a mastectomy (See Chapters 5 and 9)? This is one of the most challenging decisions and breastcancer.org lists dozens of considerations, including the size, type, grade, and location of the tumor; the degree to which it has spread; and genetic and hormonal factors. Megumi decided to have a mastectomy after cancer cells were detected at the tissue margins following a second lumpectomy.
- Should she have oncoplastic (cosmetic) surgery following a lumpectomy (see Chapter 6, p. 76)?
- Is she is a smoker, is she willing to reduce tobacco use prior to surgery and/or chemotherapy? Is she willing to reduce alcohol consumption prior to surgery and/or chemotherapy? Can you help by joining her in these efforts to increase the chances of successful treatment?
- Does she want you to help with home injections or do them herself (see Chapter 7, p. 89)?
- Does she want your assistance and the assistance of others such as friends and family with home care, transportation, or in other practical ways during her treatments (see Chapters 6–10)?
- Does she want breast reconstruction or does she prefer "going flat" (see Chapter 10, p. 143)?

- Does she want hormone therapy and, if so, what kind (see Chapter 2, p. 27)? Hormone therapy was an option presented to Megumi and she elected to begin taking Tamoxifen. Luanna's triple-negative cancer was hormone-resistant so follow-up hormone treatment after chemotherapy and a mastectomy was not an option.
- What does she want to tell family and friends and her children (see Chapters 11 and 12) about her breast cancer? How much do they need to know?
- What treatments does she want if her breast cancer is not cured with the standard treatments or if she expects that she will not recover (see Chapter 13, p. 13)? At what point might she decide that the side effects associated with ongoing treatment are compromising her quality of life and thus choose to manage her symptoms rather than continue trying new cures?

Diagnostic and Treatment Decisions

Many Decisions to Be Made During Diagnosis and Treatment

Breast cancer patients are confronted with the need to make many decisions in the course of their diagnosis and treatment. These are outlined in Box 3.1.

Decision-Making Speed

Sometimes decisions about follow-up tests and treatments need to be made quickly, as with Luanna's diagnosis of triple-negative breast cancer. Because this form is highly aggressive and potentially lethal, she started chemotherapy treatment a week after the diagnosis.

In other cases, treatment decisions can be delayed, giving her time to think it over. Megumi's initial diagnosis was for the less invasive DCIS and treatment did not start until several weeks after she received the diagnosis. But, doctors usually present treatment options with recommendations and encourage a timely decision. This is especially true in the case of advanced cancer where the treatment options are more limited, and the best decision is clear to her, as in Luanna's case. At other times, the decision is not as pressing or obvious and she may be given multiple treatment options to consider. In the latter case, it may be helpful to spend some time considering the implications of the test results and options for additional tests and treatments.

Evidence-based Decisions

Many people believe in the power of prayer, have strong faith that God or some other deity will look after them, or that what is happening to them is fate. We would never challenge such beliefs. However, we encourage the wise use of these approaches and to also consider research-based evidence that bears on the decisions that she is making. Belief in God and the power of prayer do not mean that one has to abandon seeking effective and sound medical treatments as well – they can work together. Of course, we know that the outcome of scientific research is not always correct but also considering research-based evidence can help her make decisions that are best suited for her.

How to Help Her Make Decisions

Knowing that many factors that can influence a person's choices and judgment, how can you help her make these important decisions? We have already emphasized two ways: (1) be informed about the issues that influence decisions in breast cancer treatment, and (2) encourage and help her to clarify matters in discussions with her oncology team. Remember that your role is not to unduly influence her decisions but to support her in making her own decisions. Below are some recommendations for supporting her decision-making based on the psychological literature on decision-making:

- Help her identify the factors that are most important to her. For example, it could be wanting to be around for her children, fear of recurrence of cancer, concern with possible disfigurement, concerns about side effects, or a desire for the quickest or least invasive treatment. How important are each of these factors compared to other factors for her?
- Help her examine the pros and cons of different decisions. What are the possible outcomes of the different treatment options? Making a list of pros and cons might be helpful. Remember, though, the answers to these questions are only probabilities and will not necessarily be applicable in her case.
- Help her to break down complex decisions into its parts. She doesn't have to decide about a mastectomy, reconstructive surgery, and hormone therapy all at once. Of course, they are interrelated, but considering multiple decisions and all the factors affecting them at once can be overwhelming.
- Support her if she wants to consult with family or friends. Some people find that it is helpful to get input from other family members or close friends.

- Encourage her to ask her oncology team and consult reputable sources about the evidence supporting particular options. For example, what does the research say about the relative success rate of a lumpectomy followed by radiation vs. a mastectomy for her particular type of breast cancer? What is the evidence about the increased risk of breast cancer if she stops hormone therapy? Encourage her to consult the evidence-based sources listed in this Guide, such as those at the end of Chapter 2.
- Encourage her to step away for a while before she makes a decision. If she is having trouble making a decision, and there is not a rush for medical reasons, encourage her to take some time to consider it and not make the decision right now. Encourage her to "sleep-on-it" and to reexamine her decision the next day. But encourage her as well to come to a decision within a day or so – this is cancer, after all.
- If she makes a decision remember that it is also perfectly OK for her to change her mind an hour or day later. Of course, if she is having trouble deciding and keeps changing her mind, that could even add more stress and unduly delay the decision-making process. It is important that you help her recognize what considerations she is giving most weight to and help her make the decision that she feels is the best for her so that she can begin her treatment.
- If her doctor makes a treatment recommendation, you and she should understand the basis for that recommendation before she makes a decision – never hesitate to ask for clarification. Remember the doctor is also having to make highly complex decisions.

How to Talk with Her About Decisions

How can you talk with her in a way that helps meet your goals for making the best decision? In helping her make decisions, a good strategy is to practice "active listening":

- Don't push your values on her. You may feel another lumpectomy, a mastectomy, or continued hormone therapy is best for her; or that the appearance of her breast is unimportant, but she may feel otherwise. Remember she, not you, makes the decisions.
- Don't judge, criticize, or disagree with her. As we recommended above, accept her values, concerns, thoughts, and decisions.
- Ask open-ended and nonleading questions. "How would you feel about ...?" "What are your concerns about ...?" "What is most important to you?"

- Listen carefully and reflect and paraphrase what she is saying. This may help her clarify her thoughts and communicates to her that you are listening and care. "So, it feels to you like the side effects of the hormone therapy are not worth the reductions in cancer risk?" "So, you would prefer to try another lumpectomy rather than a mastectomy because it is a less invasive surgery?"
- To help her make a decision, it is important that you understand what she is saying. If you don't understand what she is saying, more discussion might help.

How to Promote Good Communication with Her Doctor

Research has shown that good communication between her and her doctors is essential to quality health care, and good communication helps promote a positive relationship between her and those involved with her diagnosis and treatment. What you say and do during meetings with her oncology team could help or hinder effective communication between her and them. The relationship she develops with her oncology team is life-saving to her, and you and she will want these important people in her life to like her, respect her, and feel liked and valued by her. So, to respect and facilitate her relationship with her oncology team, follow these straightforward tips.

Who Does the Talking?

First, consult with her about what role she would like you to play during consultations with her oncology team. Ideally, she should be the focus of the meeting: she should be in charge of the session and ask most of the questions. She may prefer that you be a passive note-taker rather than a participant in these meetings. In this case, if she considers something to be important, it is for her to ask. Alternatively, she may prefer that you be a "backup" communicator, perhaps raising issues that she and her team members may have missed or seeking clarification when necessary. If she is experiencing high levels of anxiety or stress during the meetings and is having difficulty thinking straight or communicating her thoughts, she may prefer that you take a more active role.

Sometimes you will not know ahead of time issues what will be raised in the discussions, but it may help if she and you talk about in advance what questions she wants answered and she may have notes on these questions to remind her. Steve and Ian had different approaches to meetings with their respective oncology teams. Luanna appreciated Ian's presence and support during meetings but wanted him to trust her to pursue the areas where she wanted further clarification. Megumi initiated all the discussions with her oncology team but Steve did follow-up queries if he thought something was missed after she and the doctor finished discussing a topic.

Second Opinions About Treatment Options

We noted in Chapter 1 and in Box 3.1 that she can always ask for a second opinion before making a treatment decision. The medical profession expects this and will respect it, and virtually all care providers will present options for her to get a second opinion before making her treatment decisions. However, whenever she does this, encourage her to measure her words carefully. You want to maintain a positive relationship with her oncology team, and this is not the time for either one of you to sound challenging, critical, or to hint that the team is not doing their best for her.

Support Her to Be an Active Decision-Maker

Some patients are more passive or less expressive than others are and may be less comfortable engaging in the kind of shared decision-making between a patient and doctor that makes for the best treatment outcomes. In this case, her provider may offer patient communication skills training to help her become a more active advocate on her behalf. The skills training may include practice in sharing her feelings with the doctor, asking questions, checking understandings of information about the diagnosis and treatment, and being able to express any worries she may have about particular treatments and side effects. If she is reluctant to communicate with her oncology team and is interested, you could encourage her to attend any sessions offered by the hospital on communication skills focused on cancer issues. In the long run, being able to be her own advocate and communicate effectively with her medical team will help her make the best decisions.

Summary and Recommendations

* The diagnostic tests, their findings, and the variety of treatment options available means that critical and difficult decisions must be made, sometimes quite quickly.
* Decision-making can be stressful, especially when the consequences of the choices are very important, and you can be a source of support during these processes.

- Making objective, reasoned decisions under the stress of a serious medical condition can be difficult but there are important things we know from psychological research about how to make the best possible decisions.
- An important first step in helping her make good decisions is to understand as much as possible about the medical procedures and options.
- By asking questions and being a good listener, you can help her make the best decisions for herself.
- Treatment decisions are guided by medical aspects of her breast cancer as well as her personal values, goals, and expectations.
- By being informed and an active listener, you can help her understand the factors that the oncology team is using to recommend a particular course of action, ask questions of the team, and help her clarify her thoughts before she decides.
- You can support her if she decides to request a second opinion and help her communicate this request in a positive manner.
- The importance of evidence-based medical information in decision-making is not incompatible with your or her faith-based beliefs and her other personal principles and values.

Sources for More Information

https://en.wikipedia.org/wiki/Active_listening (a website that discusses "active listening")

Cegala, D.J., McClure, L., Marinelli, T.M., & Post, D.M. (2000). The effects of communication skills training on patients' participation during medical interviews. Patient Education and Counseling, 41:2, 209–222. 10.1002/pon.v22.12.

Lechner, B., Chow, R., Pulenzas, N., Popovic, M., Zhang, N., Zhang, X., … Merrick, J. (Eds.). (2016). Health and human development. In Cancer: Treatment, decision making and quality of life. Nova Biomedical Books. Hauppauge NY.

Li, C.-C., Matthews, A.K., Dossaji, M., & Fullam, F. (2017). The relationship of patient-provider communication on quality of life among African-American and white cancer survivors. Journal of Health Communication, 22, 584–592. 10.1080/10810730.2017.1324540

4 Detecting, Diagnosing, and Monitoring Breast Cancer

Mammograms, MRIs, Ultrasound, Echocardiograms, Electrocardiograms, and Blood Tests

Imaging techniques such as mammograms and magnetic resonance imaging (MRI) are used to detect suspicious areas in the breast that may be cancerous. Biopsies (discussed in Chapter 5) are used to examine those suspicious areas to see if they are cancer and, if so, what type of cancer. In addition, ultrasound, echocardiograms, electrocardiograms, and blood tests are used to monitor treatment progress and to detect possible side effects of the treatments.

These testing and monitoring procedures are important because their results guide decisions about what treatments might be most effective for a woman with breast cancer. To complicate these decisions, the results from these tests are sometimes unclear and different tests sometimes give conflicting results. One of those ways you can help her prepare for the tests and consider their results is to be familiar with the tests and their possible outcomes. The main purpose of this chapter is to help you understand these tests and to find the best way to support her.

This chapter first discusses some of the testing procedures that we introduced in Chapter 2 – mammograms, MRI, ultrasound, electro-cardiograms, echocardiograms, and blood tests. With that background, the chapter offers ways that you can provide emotional and practical support before, during, and after the testing.

Mammograms

Purpose

A mammogram is a low-dose X-ray of the breast that allows a specialist (radiologist) to identify suspicious areas that may be cancerous. During a

DOI: 10.4324/9781003194088-4

mammogram, the breast is exposed to small doses of X-rays that produce a computer image of the breast tissue. It cannot diagnose breast cancer – its main purpose is to see if there are any suspicious areas that warrant additional testing, such as a follow-up mammogram or biopsy.

There are differences between a regularly scheduled screening mammogram and a diagnostic mammogram. A *screening mammogram* is used for early detection of cancer in the absence of symptoms or indicators. A *diagnostic mammogram* is conducted when there are cancer symptoms or suspicious areas in the breast identified in prior mammograms. A diagnostic mammogram can involve more images and takes longer, but procedures also depend on the characteristics of the woman's breasts.

The Procedure

To prepare for the mammogram, a woman will first go through a health screening at the hospital or clinic where the mammogram will take place, if she has not already done so. The screening could include queries about current symptoms, pervious experience with mammograms and concerns, and her pregnancy status. Then, she will remove jewelry, change into a cotton gown, and remove any deodorant.

During the mammogram, a woman's breasts are compressed one at a time between two plates for several seconds while an X-ray picture is taken. Each compression takes only a few seconds but is repeated for different positions of the breast. The whole procedure takes about 15–30 minutes but can take longer for diagnostic mammograms. You can see a photo and description of the procedure at https://www.cdc.gov/cancer/breast/basic_info/mammograms.htm. An 8-minute video of the procedure can be seen at https://www.youtube.com/watch?v=175IiktUk6w. Additional descriptions of mammograms and other procedures discussed in this chapter can also be found at the sources listed at the end of this chapter.

3D Mammography

During 3D (three-dimensional) mammograms (also called breast tomosynthesis), each breast is compressed once and X-rays taken from different angles to identify suspicious areas. The images are then combined by a computer for a 3D view of the breast. 3D mammography is sometimes recommended for younger women or women with dense breast tissue, which makes traditional mammograms less effective. If a woman has dense breasts, traditional mammograms have a higher chance of missing possible cancers, or of indicating possible cancer when there is none. A recent study has also found that 3D mammography led to fewer false positives for women over 65 (https://www.breastcancer.org/symptoms/testing/types/mammograms). You can see an educational video of 3D mammography at https://www.youtube.com/watch?v=z2wuiV1_qvk. A discussion of breast density and mammography can be found at https://www.cancer.org/cancer/breast-cancer/screening-tests-and-early-detection/mammograms/breast-density-and-your-mammogram-report.html, and a more detailed and technical presentation with illustrations can be found at https://www.youtube.com/watch?v=krPxhUHTB0o.

Mammogram Results

Mammograms often provide the first indication of possible breast cancer. However, they can also lead to incorrect judgments about possible breast cancer. Factors that can affect the validity of mammogram results include the age of the woman, her weight and breast density, the quality of the mammogram picture, the size of the suspected tumor, and the skill of the radiologist. For example, some studies (see overview and references in Wikipedia/breast cancer) have found that mammograms miss about 10% of cancers, which are called *false negative results*. Mammograms can also lead to *false positive results* – when a mammogram indicates a possible cancer but there is none.

The errors have different implications, but both are important. The consequences of a false negative result are obvious and serious: The detection and treatment for her breast cancer could be delayed, thereby increasing the risk that her cancer will grow and spread and require more invasive treatments. A false positive result can cause her unnecessary worry and concern and lead to additional testing, including unnecessary biopsies.

The likelihood of false positive mammogram results is affected by several factors. They are more common in women who are younger, have dense breasts, have had breast biopsies, have breast cancer in the family, or are taking estrogen. Some research suggests that about half of all women who get an annual mammogram yearly for ten years will receive a false positive report during that time. False positive findings are especially likely for a woman's first mammogram because there are no prior mammogram results available for comparison by the radiologist.

You can read a discussion about false positive and false negative mammogram results at https://www.cancer.org/cancer/breast-cancer/screening-tests-and-early-detection/mammograms/limitations-of-mammograms.html. These sources also discuss the controversies about the relative costs (psychological, economic, health) and benefits (early detection and reduced deaths from cancer) of screening mammograms, particularly among younger women.

The images from a mammogram are examined by a radiologist who may categorize the mammogram results using the *Breast Imaging Reporting and Data System* (BI-RADS), published by the American College of Radiology. The radiologist usually informs the oncologist or woman's primary physician of the results within two weeks of the screening. As indicated in Box 4.1, the BI-RADS includes seven levels of results from a mammogram and indicates the suggested level of follow-up associated with each. Box 4.1 provides only a basic outline of the rating system and more detailed description of the BI-RADS can be found at www.cancer.org/cancer/breast-cancer/screening-tests-and-early-detection/mammograms/understanding-your-mammogram-report and at www.en.wikipedia.org/wiki/BI-RADS (which also lists several useful internet links).

An "abnormal" screening mammogram result, one indicating possible cancer such as BI-RADS Category 3–5, will likely be followed up with additional testing such as a diagnostic mammogram, ultrasound, MRI, or biopsy. After an initial screening mammogram, about 7–15% of women are called back for a second mammogram. This can be concerning but only a small percent of those who are called back will be referred for further testing or a biopsy based on findings from the second mammogram.

Magnetic Resonance Imaging

Purpose

In *breast magnetic resonance imaging* (MRI) multiple pictures are taken of the inside of the breast using radio waves and magnets. These pictures are then combined by a computer to provide a detailed image of the inside of the breast. Although MRI is sometimes used for screening if a woman has an elevated risk for breast cancer, MRI is most often used with women who have been diagnosed with breast cancer in order to locate tumors or lesions in the breast and measure their size. MRI can also be useful for further evaluation of suspicious findings from a mammogram, for presurgical screening, for the evaluation of breast implants, and to help estimate the relative benefits of a lumpectomy or mastectomy. It is not intended to replace mammogram screening because it can miss some cancers, has a high rate of false positive findings, and is more expensive.

Box 4.1   BI-RADS Categories, Definitions, and Associated Recommendations from a Mammogram

Category   Definition and Recommendation

0   Incomplete results; additional tests are needed to evaluate a
            possible abnormality
1   Negative results; no abnormality or suspicious areas identified
2   Benign structures found; no cancer was identified but possibly
            benign structures identified and regular follow-up is
            recommended
3   Likely benign structures found that require follow-up evaluation
4 (4A-4C)   Suspicious area identified and a biopsy is recommended,
            corresponding to the likelihood of being cancer
5   Highly suspicious area identified and biopsy strongly
            recommended
6   Findings on an area previously shown to be cancer; sometimes
            used to evaluate treatment outcome

Procedure

During the MRI, a woman lays prone on a flat table with an opening for her breast to extend below. She remains very still and is asked to breathe as shallowly as possible while the table slowly slides into a long narrow enclosure as her breasts are scanned. Sometimes a woman is given an injection of a solution (e.g., *gadolinium*) to help clarify the details in the breast tissue image. After the scan, the table slides out of the enclosure and the technician will remove the tube from her vein if a solution has been injected. The MRI can take as much as an hour or more, and, unlike the mammogram, no breast compression is involved. Before she leaves the MRI room, the quality of the images will be checked by a technician to see if additional imaging is needed.

The MRI involves loud clicking and clunking noises as the machine operates, so patients are given earplugs and headphones with a choice of music for distraction. Some patients are distressed by being enclosed in the tube-like enclosure for this lengthy time period without being able to move or even breathe deeply. Thus, the MRI technician will inquire if she is claustrophobic and perhaps use stress–reduction strategies, such as administration of an anxiety-reducing medication or even an earlier visit to see the machine. There is also a call button or bulb inside the machine that she can press if she becomes anxious and wants to be removed. There may be a short period of rest at the facility following the MRI if medication was used.

Discussions and illustrations of breast MRI can be found at https://www.cancer.org/cancer/breast-cancer/screening-tests-and-early-detection/breast-mri-scans.html, https://www.hopkinsmedicine.org/health/treatment-tests-and-therapies/breast-mri, and https://www.cancerresearchuk.org/about-cancer/breast-cancer/getting-diagnosed/tests-diagnose/breast-mri-scan (which includes a 1-minute video). You can see a video of breast MRIs at https://www.youtube.com/watch?v=b64 PLWO0CmA.

Results

After the breasts have been scanned and the images uploaded into a computer, a radiologist will interpret them and send a report to the woman's oncologist or primary physician. If suspicious areas are found, they will meet with the woman to review the results and discuss their implications for further testing or treatment. From the MRI scan to the report can take several days to two weeks and her doctor will inform her about when she should expect the results.

Results from the MRI can also be reported in the form of BI-RADS assessment categories, as described in Box 4.1. The results from the MRI can indicate or confirm abnormal or potentially abnormal findings, which could suggest the need for additional imaging and tests or a biopsy. The results could also be inconclusive, indicating the need for additional imaging or tests.

How You Can Help Her with a Mammogram or MRI

As you can imagine, a woman who had an MRI or has been asked to return for a follow-up diagnostic mammogram is likely to be concerned that a potential problem has been identified. Even though there is a high rate of false positives for screening mammograms and MRIs, she might feel better with some social support before and after these tests.

There are several ways you may be able to help a woman prepare for a mammogram and MRI and consider their results. As described in Box 4.2 you could help with preparation, transportation, information, and support. As always, *ask her what would be helpful*.

Box 4.2   MRI: How You Can Help Her with a Mammogram or MRI

- Educate yourself about mammograms and MRIs.
- Offer to help and ask her what would be helpful.
- Provide her with good educational material, but not so much that it becomes an overload; one or two of the sources listed at the end of this chapter should be sufficient. Remember that people differ in the amount of information they want – some want none while others will want lots of information.
- Support her decision to schedule a screening or diagnostic mammogram.
- If this is a new screening facility, remind her to bring information about previous mammograms, biopsies, and records if they are not available at the facility
- If she is at elevated risk for breast cancer, encourage her to talk to her doctor about the benefits of MRI in addition to mammograms.
- An MRI technician will carefully explain the procedures ahead of time and it might be helpful to also discuss the procedure with her, especially about her placement in the shield enclosure during the procedure. Check to see if she is comfortable with the information she has received or has additional questions. She may also want you to accompany her during this discussion.
- Remind her about preparation: Before the test, she will be asked to undress and put on a gown; metal objects, such as hair clips, jewelry, body piercings, should be removed; and she should avoid food or drinks two hours prior to the MRI. Some metal implants (e.g., implanted defibrillator or pacemaker, ear implant) preclude the use of MRI; this will be carefully evaluated by an MRI technician.
- Ask her if she would like you to accompany her or drive her to the testing facility.
- Remind her about strategies that research has found useful in reducing anxiety associated with MRIs – focus on breathing, thinking about or imagining pleasant things (guided mental imagery), listening to music, remember that she is in control

of the exam. She may also find it helpful for you or someone else to be close by during the MRI.

- It can be stressful waiting for results. If she is feeling anxious, talk to her and encourage her to talk to others if she would find that helpful. Encourage her to maintain normal social and other activities while she is waiting.
- Encourage her to contact her doctor if she hasn't received any results after two weeks.
- Help her clarify with her doctor the mammogram or MRI results and implications for additional testing or treatment. Some questions she may wish to ask if the results from imaging tests indicate the need for additional testing: (a) What other tests will follow? (b) When will they occur? (c) When will the results of those tests be available? (d) What will happen if the follow-up tests indicate cancer? (e) What will happen if the follow-up tests find a problem but it is not cancer? f) What are the costs? (g) What are the treatment implications of the MRI?

Ultrasound, Echocardiograms, and Electrocardiograms

Ultrasound

In an *ultrasound* examination, such as an echocardiogram, sound waves are used to make computer images of the inside of the breast. It is often used to look at lumps and cysts in the breast, to guide biopsies, to see how well blood is flowing inside the breast, and as a follow-up to mammograms. It can be especially useful with women who have dense breasts. During the procedure, the breast is covered with a thin gel and a wand that emits high-frequency sound waves (which we cannot hear) is moved over the skin of the breast. The sound waves bounce off breast tissue, transmitting information to a computer which produces an image of the breast. *Automated breast ultrasound* uses a larger wand to take a larger number of pictures of the entire breast. For additional information, see "Diagnosis and Monitoring of Breast Cancer, Ultrasound" in Resources at the end of this chapter. A YouTube discussions and videos of ultrasound can be found at https://www.youtube.com/watch?v=akxn2mI2rQc (2.3 minutes).

Electrocardiogram and Echocardiogram

Some treatments for breast cancer, such as chemotherapy or whole breast radiation, can affect the heart and sometimes the lungs. An electrocardiogram (EKG or ECG), echocardiogram (echo) and other heart tests are often used to examine the heart muscle, valves, or rhythm for problems before, during or after cancer treatments, particularly chemotherapy. These tests are performed in a doctor's office or at a hospital.

The tests last about five minutes to one hour, depending on whether it is an electrocardiogram or echocardiogram. First, a woman will change into a cotton gown and lie on her back or side. For the electrocardiogram, wires will be attached to electrodes placed on three or more sites in her chest area. During an echocardiogram a wand will be moved over the heart, as described in "Ultrasound."

The tests are painless and after either test, there is no recovery period and she can resume normal activities. Before scheduling the test she should inform her doctor about medications that she is taking because some of them can affect the results. Except for a few uncommon tests, she can eat and drink as usual before her EKG or echo and her doctor will inform her about any dietary restrictions. As with other imaging tests, she should wear comfortable clothing that can be removed from the waist up and avoid using lotions or powders in the chest area before the exam.

A discussion of purpose, procedures, and process of electrocardiograms can be found at https://www.cancer.net/navigating-cancer-care/diagnosing-cancer/tests-and-procedures/electrocardiogram-ekg-and-echocardiogram. A discussion and illustration of echocardiograms can be found at https://www.youtube.com/watch?v=6n2gOW5iewc.

How You Can Help

To help her you can follow most of the recommendations in Box 4.2: (1) Educate yourself about the test, (2) offer to help and ask her what would be helpful, including accompanying her to the procedure, (3) provide her with good educational material if she wishes, (4) help her understand, be comfortable with, and prepare for the procedure, (5) encourage her to maintain her normal activities and contact her doctor if she hasn't received any results after two weeks, and (6) help her clarify the results with her doctor. Hospitals and clinics differ on their policies about whether or not you can be in the room during the testing.

Blood Tests

We noted in Chapter 2 that breast cancer and chemotherapy can affect many parts of the body and that blood tests are often used to monitor a woman's overall health and especially the effects of chemotherapy. Blood tests can provide information about the number of white and red blood cells, platelets, proteins, and enzymes. This information can guide the schedule and type of chemotherapy that a woman experiences (see Chapter 7). For example, the schedule of chemotherapy sessions might be changed if a blood test indicates possible liver or kidney damage. In Megumi's case, chemotherapy sessions were stopped for two weeks when blood tests indicated possible damage to her liver. They were resumed when ALT (see below) measures indicated improvement in her liver function.

Her doctor will explain the meaning of the blood tests and many cancer treatment centers have websites that explain them. A few of the more common blood tests used during chemotherapy are outlined in Box 4.3.

A brief description of blood test results and their implications can be found at https://www.cancer.org/treatment/understanding-your-diagnosis/tests/understanding-your-lab-test-results.html.

Blood Marker Tests are used to identify circulating cancer cells and proteins that serve as markers for cancer. Sometimes, cells break off from the tumor and move into the blood stream. Blood markers are identified through simple blood tests that can be done before treatment to help

---

Box 4.3   Blood Tests Used during Chemotherapy

- *Complete blood count (CBC)* – measures the number and quality of white blood cells, red blood cells, and platelets. A CBC is done to check her general health and to monitor changes in her health during treatment.
- *Blood urea nitrogen (BUN)* and creatinine – measures how well her kidneys are working.
- *Alanine aminotransferase (ALT)* and aspartate transaminase (AST) – measure how well her liver is working and to see if the cancer has spread to the liver.
- *Alkaline phosphatase* – measures how well her liver is working and to see if the cancer has spread to the liver or the bone.

diagnose the breast cancer and later to determine whether the cancer has moved to other parts of the body. Blood marker tests are described at: https://www.breastcancer.org/symptoms/testing/types/blood_marker. Blood tests are familiar to most people: the patient sits in a chair with the arm resting, sometimes a band is placed around the arm to help the nurse or technician (called a phlebotomist) locate a vein, the area is swabbed with an anesthetic, a needle is inserted, and vials of blood are withdrawn. The needle is then withdrawn, a bandage placed over the site (usually a small piece of gauze held in place by paper tape), and the vials are labeled and sent for analysis. Most patients can then leave and resume normal activities.

Summary and Recommendations

This chapter provided basic information about mammograms, breast MRIs, ultrasound, EKG, and blood tests and suggested ways to help a woman undergoing these assessments.

- A mammogram uses X-rays to examine suspicious areas in a breast. It cannot diagnose breast cancer but can indicate the need for additional testing. The procedure involves compression of the breasts while X-rays are taken, and results are often communicated with a BI-RADS assessment system. 3D mammography is sometimes recommended for women with dense breast tissue.
- In a breast MRI, radio waves are used to take multiple pictures of the inside of the breast. MRIs are sometimes used for screening when there is an elevated risk for breast cancer and are often used with women who have already been diagnosed with breast cancer. During an MRI, a woman will lie prone on a flat table while the table slides into a shield enclosure where her breasts are scanned.
- Mammography and MRI are useful screening and monitoring, but both can give false results.
- Blood tests are often used to monitor the effects and possible side effects of chemotherapy and to evaluate a woman's overall health.
- Offer to help and ask her what would be helpful, such as accompanying her to the appointments, help with preparing for the exams, providing sources of information, or discussing the procedure and results with her doctor.
- Be informed and provide her with good educational material if she would like.
- Provide emotional and practical support for her during stressful aspects of the process.

- Support her if she decides to ask for a second opinion about the results of any test.

Sources for More Information

Diagnosis and Monitoring

https://www.cancer.ca/en/cancer-information/cancer-type/breast/diagnosis/?region=on#:~:text=Blood%20chemistry%20tests%20used%20to%20stage%20breast%20cancer,may%20check%20it%20again%20during%20or%20after%20treatment. (Discusses many diagnostic and monitoring procedures in breast cancer, including mammography, ultrasound, biopsies, and blood tests).

Mammograms

https://www.cdc.gov/cancer/breast/basic_info/mammograms.htm (basic information)
https://www.youtube.com/watch?v=175IiktUk6w (an 8-minute video of the procedure)
https://www.cancer.org/cancer/ breast-cancer/screening-tests-and-early-detection/mammograms/breast-den-sity-and-your-mammogram-report.html (a discussion of mammograms, breast density, and interpreting the results of a mammogram).
https://www.youtube.com/watch?v=krPxhUHTB0o (a more detailed and technical presentation of mammograms with illustrations).

MRI

https://www.cancer.org/cancer/breast-cancer/screening-tests-and-early-detection/breast-mri-scans.html (discussions and illustrations of breast MRI)
https://www.cancerresearchuk.org/about-cancer/breast-cancer/getting-diagnosed/tests-diagnose/breast-mri-scan (discussions and illustrations of breast MRI, also includes a 1-minute video)
https://www.youtube.com/watch?v=b64PLWO0CmA (videos of breast MRIs)

Ultrasound

https://www.youtube.com/watch?v=akxn2mI2rQc (YouTube discussions and videos of ultrasound 2.3 minutes) https://www.youtube.com/watch?v=yEEofwP-8eo (YouTube discussions and videos of ultrasound 1.1 minute)

EKG (or ECG) and Echo

https://www.cancer.net/navigating-cancer-care/diagnosing-cancer/tests-and-procedures/electrocardiogram-ekg-and-echocardiogram. https://www.youtube.com/watch?v=6n2gOW5iewc (a discussion and illustration of echocardiograms)

Blood Markers

https://www.breastcancer.org/symptoms/testing/types/blood_marker (a discussion of blood tests during breast cance r treatment)

5 Biopsies

Mammograms and other imaging methods described in Chapter 4 can help identify areas of the breast that might contain cancer cells. However, these methods cannot determine if the cells in the suspicious area are benign or malignant. To determine if the cells are cancerous, a *biopsy* is needed. There are several types of biopsies, described in Box 5.1, but all involve using a needle to remove a small amount of breast tissue or fluid that is then examined under a microscope by a pathologist. The findings from the biopsy are then reported to the patient's primary care provider.

Information about biopsies is included in most books on breast cancer, on many websites, and many clinics and hospitals have printed information and videos about biopsies that a woman can access before the procedure. We have also included sources of information on biopsies at the end of this chapter. This chapter describes different types of biopsies, biopsy procedures, their possible results, the risks and benefits of biopsies, and their side effects. The chapter emphasizes ways you can help before, during, and after a biopsy.

Types of Biopsies

As described in Box 5.1, there are several types of biopsies, but all involve the removal of a small section of tissue or fluid from the breast for examination. The type of biopsy depends on the size, location, and appearance of the suspicious area and the woman's medical condition and history. It is important for her to understand the type of biopsy that will be performed and, as we stressed in Chapter 2, you can help ensure that she gets complete information from her doctor about the procedures, its risks, and benefits.

You can see from Box 5.1 that the types of biopsies differ in their procedures and their degree of invasiveness: Fine needle aspiration, core needle aspiration, vacuum-assisted biopsy, and stereotactic biopsy are the

DOI: 10.4324/9781003194088-5

Box 5.1 Types of Biopsies

- *Fine needle biopsy (fine needle aspiration, FNA)* involves the use of a very fine needle and syringe to remove cells or fluid from a suspicious area. It is often used when a tumor cannot be felt.
- Core needle biopsy involves the insertion of a small hollow needle to obtain a small number of cells from a suspicious area for examination. This needle can remove a larger sample than can a fine needle biopsy and is sometimes inserted several times to remove multiple samples. Local anesthesia is usually used and the process is often guided by ultrasound, mammogram, or MRI. It takes 30–60 minutes.
- *Vacuum-assisted core biopsy* is similar to a core needle and involves a suction device to remove fluid and cells.
- *Stereotactic core needle biopsy* uses a special instrument to guide the needle.
- *Ultrasound-guided biopsy* uses sound waves to locate the tumor or other suspicious area. Biopsies can also be guided by *magnetic resonance imaging*.
- *Wire localization* uses a small wire that is inserted into the breast to help the surgeon locate the suspicious area.
- *Surgical (excision) biopsy* involves the surgical removal of all or part of a suspicious lump. It can involve open *excision biopsy* to remove an entire lump, *sentinel node biopsy* to remove a lymph node, or *axillary node dissection* to remove multiple lymph nodes. It is sometimes done with local anesthesia but a light general anesthesia may be used. Surgical biopsies are often done in a hospital's outpatient clinic.
- *Liquid/fluid biopsy* was approved by the FDA in the fall of 2020 and involves the diagnosis and monitoring of cancer based on blood samples. It is less invasive that needle biopsies, can be used more often with little discomfort, and may be useful for early diagnosis and to monitor treatment effects.
- *Punch skin biopsy* is used to sample affected cells in the skin surrounding the breast or nipples. It is performed in a surgeon's office with a local anesthetic.

least invasive forms. They are usually associated with less pain and scaring, less risk of infection, and a shorter time to recovery. These differences emphasize the importance of finding out ahead of time the type of biopsy that will be performed, what the effects might be, and what post-biopsy care might be needed.

Sentinel Lymph Node Biopsy

If she has been diagnosed with breast cancer, it is important to know how far the cancer has spread and the lymphatic system is the first place cancer cells often spread to. The lymphatic system is composed of tissues, organs, and lymphatic vessels that are similar to veins and capillaries of the circulatory system except that they circulate lymph fluid. The lymph vessels are connected to lymph nodes, which are small round glands that filter and attack harmful substances such as cancer cells and infections that are carried in through the lymph fluid. There are hundreds of lymph nodes in the body, and some are under the arm and close to the breast. Cancer cells in the breast can break away from a tumor and travel through the lymphatic system, and the first place they can spread to is the lymph nodes under the arm. The number of lymph nodes with cancer helps determine the stage of breast cancer (see p. 18, Chapter 2).

If cancer cells have been detected in a breast biopsy and the lymph nodes are swollen or appear abnormal in an ultrasound, a surgeon might remove a small piece of one or more lymph nodes under the arm closest to the breast with a needle biopsy (see Box 5.1). That small sample will be examined under a microscope to see if the cancer has spread. If cancer cells are detected, one or more sentinel lymph nodes will be surgically removed during a lumpectomy or mastectomy and further examined.

The *sentinel lymph nodes* are the first lymph nodes that receive lymph fluid from around a breast tumor and the first to which cancer cells are likely to spread from a breast tumor; there can be more than one sentinel lymph node. If breast cancer has been confirmed in the sentinel lymph nodes, other lymph nodes might also be removed (referred to as axillary lymph node dissection) to gather more information about the possible spread of cancer.

A sentinel lymph node biopsy might be performed before or after a tumor is surgically removed during a lumpectomy or mastectomy (see Chapters 6 and 9). In the latter case the entire lymph node will be removed and sent for microscopic examination. In cases where chemotherapy precedes a mastectomy, a fine needle biopsy is sometimes used to determine if the sentinel nodes should also be removed during the surgery.

The results of a sentinel node biopsy are important for treatment planning. The medical oncologist will discuss treatment options and whether additional lymph nodes should be removed. If no cancer cells have been detected in the sentinel nodes, it is unlikely that the cancer has spread. The results can indicate whether additional lymph node surgery and radiation therapy after a lumpectomy or mastectomy will be needed. In some cases, the sentinel node can be examined during the surgery to see if more lymph nodes should be removed right away, negating the necessity of her coming back for additional lymph node surgery.

https://www.cancer.org/cancer/breast-cancer/treatment/surgery-for-breast-cancer/lymph-node-surgery-for-breast-cancer.html discusses sentinel lobe biopsies.

The Biopsy Procedure

Biopsies are considered surgical procedures and can take place in hospitals, clinics, or a doctor's office, usually on an outpatient basis. The exact procedure will depend on the type of biopsy and the hospital or clinic where it occurs. Her doctor should inform her ahead of time about procedures, and she will probably be advised to stop all blood thinners such as aspirin for up to a week or two before the biopsy to reduce the chance of excessive bleeding.

Fine needle and core biopsies are often done in a doctor's office with only local anesthesia to numb the breast area. Needle placement in biopsies is often guided by ultrasound (see below and p. 51 in Chapter 4). The needle is so thin that injection of an anesthetic may hurt more than the biopsy. For a sentinel node biopsy, the surgeon often injects a small amount of dye or radioactive solution to identify the sentinel node. Removal of the sentimental nodes usually occurs under general anesthesia.

In most cases, she will arrive an hour or more before the procedure and after checking in will change into a hospital gown. Her clothing and belongings will be stored, so she should bring only those that are important (no jewelry, money, etc.) and wear comfortable clothes. She can store all of her belongings in a locker in the pre-operation area or you can keep her more valuable items while you are waiting for her. After she has changed, the doctor and nurses will check her identity and the purpose of the visit to avoid mistaken identities or procedures and to ensure she understands and consents to the procedures (this is similar to the safety interview and consent process done for all surgical procedures). She should inform them about any allergies and medications or supplements she is taking and about any recent illnesses. A needle might then be inserted into a vein in her arm and taped down to administer medication to help her relax. If she has received medication to help her relax, she will need a little recovery time and a ride home.

Most biopsies are performed with local anesthesia and sometimes with a light general anesthesia or medications to help the woman relax during the procedure. The procedure takes only a few minutes, and she will likely be awake during it. In the surgery room, she will be given a local anesthetic to numb the skin and she will probably feel only some slight pressure when the needle is inserted. It is usually painless, but some women report being sensitive to the procedure. For small areas, the needle placement can be guided by an ultrasound or other imaging methods. In these cases, the surgeon will monitor the placement of the needle on a screen during the procedure. The surgeon may also a use a tiny wire to help guide the biopsy needle to the right spot in the breast. Sometimes, multiple samples of breast tissue will be taken. The entire process can take 30–60 minutes, but the actual tissue extraction takes only a few minutes. A video of an ultrasound-guided biopsy can be found at:

www.radiologyinfo.org/en/info.cfm?pg=breastbius (describes ultrasound-guided biopsies).

www.cancer.org/cancer/breast-cancer/screening-tests-and-early-detection/breast-biopsy/core-needle-biopsy-of-the-breast.html (describes core needle aspiration).

www.cancer.gov/about-cancer/diagnosis-staging/staging/sentinel-node-biopsy-fact-sheet (describes sentinel node biopsies).

www.youtube.com/watch?v=ink1nyRCnDQ (illustrates the biopsy process).

After the biopsy procedure, she will walk or be taken to a recovery room, depending on the anesthesia used. After a short rest, she will change back into her normal clothes and collect her personal effects. Recovery time is usually short, depending on the medication she was administered.

After the biopsy she may be provided with a special protective bra, a small bandage, and possibly an antibiotic medication over the biopsy site. Stitches are not usually required but are possible with more invasive procedures. A member of the surgery team will let her know how to bathe, when to change any bandages, and when to come back to the clinic. It will be helpful to have written instructions about how to take care of the biopsy site, including any needed bandaging instructions so that you could assist with this later, if she wishes.

Interpreting the Results

Sometimes, the most difficult part of a biopsy is waiting for the results. As you can appreciate, it would be natural for her to worry about the outcome of a biopsy, even though about 80% of the results from biopsies in the USA show no sign of breast cancer. This contrasts with higher rates of positive findings in some other countries where the criteria for who should get a biopsy are more stringent. It will be helpful for both of you to maintain your usual positive social interactions, interests, and activities while waiting for results.

If the pathologist identifies the suspicious area as cancer, they can also indicate whether the cells are noninvasive or are invasive and can spread to other parts of the body. The pathology report can also indicate the type of cancer and grade it from low to high, which can indicate the seriousness of the cancer and the likelihood of successful treatment – lower grade cancers have a better prognosis, as discussed in Chapter 2, Boxes 2.1–2.3. The pathologist examines the size and shape of the cells and their nucleus, how the cells are arranged, and their rate of dividing. Pathologists commonly stain the cells to help identify their type and source of the cancer cells. For biopsies of tissues removed during a lumpectomy (see Chapter 6, p. 24), the report will also indicate if cancer cells were detected at the edges (margins) of the tissue that was removed. Biopsy results can also specify if the cancer is affected by certain hormones, which indicate whether or not hormone therapy might be beneficial for treating the cancer (see Box 2.3).

Sometimes, the results of a biopsy are unclear, and her doctor may recommend another biopsy. More detailed information about pathology reports can be found at https://www.cancer.gov/about-cancer/diagnosis-staging/diagnosis/pathology-reports-fact-sheet#what-information-does-a-pathology-report-usually-include.

Even if a breast tumor is judged to be benign and unlikely to spread, some types can still indicate she has a higher risk of developing breast cancer in the future. In addition, a diagnosis of some types of cancers may indicate the need for genetic testing for gene mutations that could put her and close family members at risk for both breast and ovarian cancer now and in the future. Routine screening is especially important in this case (see Chapter 2, p. 45).

Risks and Negative Aspects

It is understandable for her to be anxious about a procedure that involves sticking a needle into her breast and removing tissue. That is why anxiety-reducing medication may be administered just prior to the procedure. You can also help by suggesting some of the relaxation methods described in Chapter 14.

Breast biopsies are relatively safe, but some risks include infection, swelling, bruising, mild pain, and bleeding. Her doctor will discuss post-biopsy care with her. You can help by taking notes if there is no handout available. Over-the-counter medication is usually sufficient to reduce any pain, but for several days she should avoid pain medications that list aspirin as the active ingredient because it is a blood "thinner" that can increase the risk of bleeding. She should also wait a few days before resuming strenuous exercise.

One unlikely complication of sentinel node biopsy is lymphedema – fluid buildup and swelling because the lymph vessels can't adequately drain lymph fluid from the breast or arm area. Sentinel node biopsy reduces the chance of lymphedema because only one or a few lymph nodes are removed.

How You Can Help

After the biopsy and before you leave, be clear about any instructions regarding care of the biopsy site. Biopsies are relatively safe and significant side effects are rare, but you can help her look out for possible negative effects, especially swelling, redness, fluid buildup, fever, chills, or other signs of infection. With any sign of infection, encourage her to call her doctor right away.

You can also help by being knowledgeable about the procedure, it's possible findings and risks, post-biopsy care, and by being empathic and understanding. Remember that some people like lots of information about medical procedures and others would rather not be told too much about them. Also, some people find social support for medical procedures helpful while others would prefer to cope with them alone. As always, offer to help and ask her what would be helpful – let her preferences guide your level and type of support and education.

The results of the biopsy can be difficult to understand, especially for someone under stress about the procedure, the findings, and their implications. In her 2017 book on breast cancer, Margaret Lesh said "it's so important to have an advocate with you. An observer, another ear – for any kind of important medical decisions. Don't go by yourself if you can help it. Sometimes it's hard to process information that is thrown at you during an especially stressful time" (pg. 32).

As we discussed in Chapter 3, if she would like support, do your best to always go along or have a friend or family member accompany her, so

Box 5.2   How You Can Help Her

- Offer to help and ask her what would be helpful.
- Serve as her advocate in discussions with her doctor about any aspect of the biopsy process and its results. She should be able to get a copy of the report. You can help her understand:

  a   The type of biopsy and exact procedure and why that type was selected; an examination of the mammogram to pinpoint the biopsy site might be helpful.

  b   How long it will take and how long she will be in the clinic or hospital.

  c   If will it be painful and will an anesthetic be used.

  d   In what part of the breast or arm the biopsy will occur.

  e   How the suspicious area will be located.

  f   If there will be scarring or other negative side effects of the procedure, such as bruising or discomfort.

  g   What are the risks and possible side effects.

  h   How to care for herself after the procedure or what precautious should she take; can she shower, remove any bandages.

  i   If it will limit her activities, such as exercise, work, school, and childcare; will she feel tired.

  j   How long until she receives the results and how will she receive them.

  k   If the results are final or will another biopsy be required.

  l   When the follow-up appointment is scheduled.

  m   How much it will cost (this could be a co-pay only or full payment for some procedures, depending on her insurance policy)

- Take a copy of this box with you when she consults with her doctor – this is a long list of questions.
- Read about biopsies so that you can help her get complete information on the specific biopsy procedure from her doctor.
- Remind her about preparations for the biopsy –

  a   Avoid aspirin and other blood thinners up to a week or more prior to the biopsy.

  b   Wear loose clothing and bring only necessary items.

  c   No deodorant, lotions, creams, etc. on the breast or under the arm.

d   Ensure the doctor is aware of health and pregnancy status and any allergies.

- Drive her to and from the biopsy or arrange for someone else to do this; this is especially important if she receives any general anesthesia or medication to help her relax during the procedure.
- Help her monitor any side effects such as swelling, redness, or any other signs of infection; remind her about other post-biopsy care, such as bathing, care of bandages, and follow-up appointments.
- Help her understand the results if the findings indicate cancer: Invasive or noninvasive? Spreading? Will it respond to hormone therapy? What stage is it? Treatment implications?
- Encourage her to call her doctor if she has any concerns or if there are signs of infections.
- Know the phone number of who to call if there are serious side effects or concerns.
- Help her procure over-the-counter medication she may need for pain, such as an alternative pain medication that does not contain aspirin.
- Help her stay active and relaxed while waiting for the results of the biopsy.
- Engage others to provide practical and emotional support.

you or someone else can be there during the discussions and help clarify anything that is unclear – serve as her advocate, if she would find that helpful. Remember some people are reluctant to question their doctor, and some will not have thought about important questions to ask. You could help her prepare a list of questions before this meeting so that neither of you has to try to remember what to ask at a time when she may be hearing lots of new and sometimes confusing information. Box 5.2 lists some questions to ask before and after a biopsy.

If the biopsy indicates cancer, the meeting with the doctor to go over the biopsy report is a time to begin making important decisions, as we discussed in Chapter 3. This is the time when she and her doctor will discuss what comes next: more tests or the beginning of treatment, and which treatment. Chapter 3 discusses many ways that you can help her be clear about the potential risks and benefits of the next step.

A pathology report indicating cancer cells will be more understandable if you help her to make certain the doctor has explained the type and size of the tumor, whether it is invasive or noninvasive and growing, and other information that affects treatment decisions. She should understand the next possible steps and the reasons for them so that she can make the decision that is best for her. Think about what *you* would want to know before making such a decision!

Sometimes, she or her doctor might wish a second opinion. In that case, samples of the tissue that the pathologist examined must be provided for that second opinion. Many facilities offer second opinions: the National Cancer Institutes are often a good source of options for a second opinion. You can help in the discussion about the need for a second opinion and help locate facilities that provide second opinions; see.

https://www.cancer.org/treatment/finding-and-paying-for-treatment/choosing-your-treatment-team/seeking-a-second-opinion.html

Summary and Recommendations

- There are several types of needle or surgical biopsies, but all involve the removal and microscopic examination of tissue, cells, or fluids to determine if the suspicious cells are benign or malignant.
- To see if the cancer has spread beyond the breast, one or more lymph nodes under the arm may also be examined if cancer cells were detected in the breast biopsy.
- Biopsies are usually done on an outpatient basis and can occur in hospitals, clinics, or a doctor's office.
- Sometimes medication is administered to help a woman relax before a biopsy, and the exact biopsy procedure will depend on the type of biopsy performed.
- For most biopsies, she will be awake during the procedure, which takes only a few minutes.
- Some sentinel lymph node biopsies are performed with a needle biopsy with local anesthesia. In others, the sentinel node is surgically removed while the woman is under general anesthesia
- The biopsy sample is sent to a pathologist for microscopic examination who will then send a pathology report to her primary care doctor.
- The biopsy report will indicate whether the tissue or cells are cancerous or noncancerous. If cancerous, the report will indicate other aspects of the cancer that can be used to guide treatment.
- Biopsies are relatively safe and significant side effects of biopsies are rare, but it is important to monitor for any signs of infection.
- If she would like your assistance, you can serve as her advocate in discussions with her doctors and help her understand biopsy results

and make decisions about future testing and treatment. Remember these are her decisions!

- Help her prepare for the biopsy and drive her to and from the clinic.
- Help monitor any side effects and encourage her to call her doctor if there are any signs of infection or other serious side effects.
- Encourage her to maintain her usual activities while waiting for biopsy results.
- Engage others to provide practical and social support, if she would find this helpful.

Sources for More Information

https://www.amazon.com/Let-Get-This-Off-Chest-ebook/dp/B00DQSV-L4W (a book by Lesh, M. (2013). Let me get this off my chest: A breast cancer survivor over-shares.)

https://www.nationalbreastcancer.org/breast-cancer-biopsy (includes a video discussion of three types of biopsies)

https://www.cancer.net/cancer-types/breast-cancer/diagnosis (discusses imaging and biopsies)

https://www.cancer.gov/about-cancer/diagnosis-staging/diagnosis/pathology-reports-fact-sheet (discusses the pathology report from a biopsy)

https://www.breastcancer.org/symptoms/testing/types/biopsy (discusses the biopsy procedure)

https://www.youtube.com/watch?v=SC6ZAClF59c (a video of an ultrasound guided biopsy)

https://www.cancer.gov/about-cancer/diagnosis-staging/staging/sentinel-node-biopsy-fact-sheet (describes sentinel node biopsy)

6 Lumpectomies and Breast-Sparing Surgery

Breast cancer is almost always treated surgically, and a *lumpectomy* is the least invasive form of surgery to treat breast cancer. Different terms, such as *breast-conserving surgery*, *wide local excision*, or *excisional biopsy* are sometimes used to refer to the same surgical process as a "lumpectomy." The National Cancer Institute labels a "lumpectomy," "partial mastectomy," "breast-conserving surgery," and "segmental mastectomy" as similar words to describe "breast-sparing surgery."

In breast-sparing surgeries, such as a lumpectomy, only the part of the breast containing the cancer is removed, which allows the woman to keep most of her breast. This is in contrast to a mastectomy (Chapter 9) where the entire breast, or major portions of the breast, is removed. In a lumpectomy, a small section of the tissue surrounding the cancer is also removed to ensure that all the cancer has been taken out and to check if any cancer cells remain at the edges (margins) of the removed tissue.

The goal of this chapter is to provide you with an understanding of lumpectomies, their effects, and side effects so you can better help her before, during, and after the surgery. This chapter describes what happens during a lumpectomy, how she should prepare for it, possible results, potential side effects, and how to cope with those side effects. The next section discusses the circumstances in which a lumpectomy is a viable option. We also discuss how you can help her prepare for a lumpectomy and promote her post-lumpectomy recovery.

Choosing Between a Lumpectomy or Mastectomy

In Chapter 3, we note that an important treatment decision a woman must sometimes make is whether to have breast-conserving surgery or a mastectomy after a positive biopsy reveals she has breast cancer. Box 2.4 (p. 26) describes the types of breast cancer surgery.

DOI: 10.4324/9781003194088-6

Her doctor will explain the risks and benefits of each surgical option and may recommend a lumpectomy if her particular type and stage of cancer – along with consideration of other factors – makes this a viable option for her. Depending on her diagnosis and additional relevant information, her doctor may instead offer her the choice between a lumpectomy or mastectomy, or recommend a mastectomy.

Another situation that requires her to choose from surgical options is when cancer cells have been identified at the margins of the tissue sample after the first or second lumpectomy. Megumi chose a mastectomy, rather than a third lumpectomy, after cancer cells were found at the margins in both her first and second lumpectomies.

We noted in Chapter 3 that treatment decisions can be influenced by many factors in addition to the characteristics of the cancer. These include a woman's family history of cancer, evidence of genetic mutations, the importance to her of the appearance of the breast and her feelings about disfigurement, and concerns about possible recurrence of her breast cancer or the development of new cancers.

A lumpectomy, rather than a mastectomy, is sometimes selected as the first surgical treatment, depending on the size of the tumor, the size of the tumor relative to breast size, and the number of tumors that have been identified. Lumpectomies are often the treatment of choice when the cancer is small, early stage, or in certain precancerous states such as DCIS (see p. 19 in Chapter 2). The American Cancer Society (https:// www.cancer.org/cancer/breast-cancer/treatment/surgery-for-breast-cancer/ breast-conserving-surgery-lumpectomy.html) lists dozens of considerations, including the size, type, grade, and location, of the tumor; its genetic traits; and rate of growth. Some of these factors are outlined in Box 3.1 (p. 37).

A lumpectomy is often followed by chemotherapy (see Chapter 7), radiation treatment (see Chapter 8), and hormone therapy to reduce the chance of recurrence (see Chapter 7). If the cancer is triple-negative (i.e., it is not fueled by estrogen, progesterone, or the HER2 protein), however, hormone therapy cannot be used.

If the doctor makes a treatment recommendation, you and she should understand the basis for that decision – never hesitate to ask and to discuss with her doctor all factors that are important to her in deciding what to choose. As we suggested in Chapter 3, it may help to take some time to consider the decision if surgical treatment is not immediately necessary. However, remember that delays in treatment could have negative consequences for her health.

Preparing for a Lumpectomy

The necessary steps to prepare for a lumpectomy are similar to those for a biopsy (Chapter 5) and differ across clinics and the type of lumpectomy that is to be performed. If she decides to have a lumpectomy, it will likely be scheduled soon after a positive biopsy finding. If the lump is too small to feel, the precise area to be removed may have been identified by a small marker or guided by a thin wire placed there during an earlier biopsy.

She will meet with her oncologist, surgeon, or other member of the oncology team before the lumpectomy to discuss the procedure and how to prepare for it. There will be a lot of information to absorb during this discussion, so she may like your help to be sure she understands the preparation, procedure, and its risks. If she would like you to accompany her, take a copy of Box 6.1 and take notes, or make recordings if allowed, about the answers to questions that are important to her.

When talking with her doctors, be sure you both understand the procedure, how to prepare for it, its risks and benefits, and post-lumpectomy care. She will most likely be given written instructions with much of this information, and it can be useful to review these before you leave; ask the nurse or doctor if something isn't clear to you. For legal reasons, consent forms are required to list all possible risks including those that are extremely rare.

She should take time to completely understand the procedure and its risks. A lumpectomy is a common surgical procedure, and severe complications following lumpectomies are rare (less than 1 per 100,000–200,000). If you are with her, assume that you are going through the procedure – what would you want to know? You and she can select some of the items in Box 6.1 that are most important to her as good starting places for the discussions. Many of the questions are probably addressed in written material provided by the hospital and can also be answered by a member of the oncology team. You may have talked about some of them when deciding whether or not to have a lumpectomy. She may be called before the surgery to remind her about some of these issues, such as the time for her arrival at the hospital and how to prepare for the lumpectomy.

As with a biopsy, she will be advised when to stop all blood thinners, such as aspirin, and some vitamins and herbs before the lumpectomy to reduce the chance of excessive bleeding during surgery. Smoking and excessive alcohol also introduce risks so should be avoided at this time. She should tell the doctor about any vitamins, medications, or supplements she is taking. The purpose of this information is to identify anything that might interfere with the effectiveness of the surgery.

Box 6.1   Questions to Ask Her Oncology Nurse or Doctor About the Lumpectomy

Questions About the Lumpectomy Procedures

- What kind of anesthesia will be used, and when will be it administered? Will it be local (regional) or general, or both?
- How will the surgeon locate the cancer that is to be removed?
- How will the surgeon know if all of the cancer was removed?
- How will the surgeon decide how much tissue needs to be removed?
- Will underarm lymph nodes also be removed?
- How long will the surgery take, and how long will she be in recovery?

Questions About What Happens After the Lumpectomy

- What if cancer cells are detected at the margins of the tissue removed?
- When will she get the biopsy results from the lumpectomy?
- Will she go home with a surgical drain?
- Will there be scaring, bruising, or discomfort?
- Will it change the look of her breast?
- What are the risks, side effects, and possible complications?
- Will there be a risk for lymphedema (excess fluid causing swelling, edema) after surgery?
- Will she need to stay at the clinic or hospital after the surgery?
- When will she receive the results and how will they be communicated to her?
- Will radiation treatments, chemotherapy, or hormone therapy follow the lumpectomy? If so, when and for how long?

If she would like, you can help by marking the surgery date on a calendar, including when she should begin precautions, such as stopping any non-essential medications and stop taking aspirin. You could also gently remind her about preparations, such as those outlined in Box 6.2, the day before the surgery.

In most cases, she will be told to arrive two or more hours before the surgery. After checking in and going through pretesting (which, at the time of this writing, included a test for the COVID-19 virus), she will be

---

Box 6.2   Preparations for the Lumpectomy (confirm with her surgeon or other sources of information about these)

- Avoid aspirin and other blood thinners prior to the lumpectomy, for the number of days recommended by her doctor
- Wear loose clothing and bring only necessary items
- No deodorant, lotions, creams, etc. on the breast or under the arm
- Ensure that the doctor is aware of health and pregnancy status and any allergies
- No food or drink 12 hours before the lumpectomy
- Arrive on time
- Arrange for a ride home

---

escorted to a preoperative room and change into a hospital gown. Her effects will be stored, so remind her to bring only those she needs (no jewelry, money, etc.) and to wear comfortable clothes. She may appreciate your holding her cellphone and some personal effects for her while she undergoes pretesting and surgery.

After she has changed, the doctor and nurses will question her about her identity and purpose of the visit to avoid mistaken identities or procedures and to ensure she understands and consents to the procedures. She may also speak to an anesthesiologist who will ask about her medical history and prior experiences with anesthesia. Usually, you can remain with her during these conversations and help her ask questions and clarify any issues that arise. During one of these visits, her breast may be marked with a felt tipped pen to show which breast will receive the lumpectomy to avoid any mistakes. In some cases a mammogram or ultrasound may be used before the surgery to identify and mark the tumor with a radioactive substance or thin wire, so that it can be precisely located during the surgery.

A needle may be inserted in a hand or arm vein by a nurse to administer medications to help her relax prior to and during the lumpectomy. Relaxation strategies described in Chapter 14 may also help.

She will be asked about any allergies and medications or supplements that she is taking and about any recent illnesses. After these preparations, she will be assisted into an operation room for the lumpectomy. Most clinics would allow you to be with her during these preparations up to the time she leaves the preoperative room. If in doubt, ask. After she is assisted into the operating room, you will be in a waiting area until she has recovered from the operation. If she has been under general anesthesia, she will first go to a recovery room until she is fully conscious. Depending on the clinic and circumstances, you might be permitted to wait for her in the recovery room or join her after she becomes conscious.

What Happens During a Lumpectomy

Because the procedures vary across clinics and the type of lumpectomy, it is important to clarify exactly what will happen before, during, and after the lumpectomy. Many clinics and hospitals supply written documents to outline the whole process, but she may still have questions. Remember she may feel anxious about the lumpectomy or hesitant to ask the doctor specific questions – if she would find it helpful, you can serve as her advocate and help her get information and answers to her questions. Some aspects to clarify about the lumpectomy are listed in Box 6.1.

Before the surgery she will be assisted to the surgical room, positioned on a surgical table, and hooked up with various devices to monitor vital signs such as blood pressure, heart rate, breathing, and blood oxygen. The lumpectomy will be performed under either general anesthetic or a local anesthetic, depending on the type of lumpectomy and the practice followed by the hospital or clinic that performs it. If she is awake, she will likely feel only a slight tugging sensation. After the surgery, the incision will be closed, usually with stitches that will dissolve or be removed at a later time by her doctor or a nurse.

The tissue that was removed will be sent to a pathologist who examines it for the presence of any cancer cells left behind at the edges of the excised tissue and to provide more information about the tumor (see also Chapter 5). If it has "positive margins," meaning more cancerous cells were found at the edges of the sample, the doctor may recommend another lumpectomy or a mastectomy, as we discussed earlier.

What to Expect After a Lumpectomy

Recovery

Most lumpectomies are performed on an outpatient basis, so she can probably return home after resting for a short period in a recovery room. During this time, her vital signs will be monitored, and she will be able to leave once her condition is stable and she feels able to leave. Most likely, you can be with her during this time. Besides offering emotional support and helping her understand post-operation instructions, she will need someone to drive her home.

Although a lumpectomy is generally an outpatient procedure, she may be scheduled to stay overnight if her lymph nodes were removed (*sentinel lymph node biopsy* or *axillary lymph node dissection;* see Chapter 5) or if she is experiencing pain or bleeding. If she lives far from the surgical site, some clinics will arrange transportation services and overnight accommodations.

Post-lumpectomy Care

Most clinics provide written instructions about care in the days and weeks following the lumpectomy. The instructions will detail how to care for the surgical site and dressing, and include advice regarding bathing and showering, use of pain medication, exercising, and any signs of infection to watch for.

She and a member of her oncology team will probably discuss post-lumpectomy care and review any written instructions. Someone on the team will confirm the follow-up appointment before she leaves the recovery room. You and she should be clear about post-surgery care before the lumpectomy and again before she leaves the clinic after the surgery (Box 6.3). If you have any questions, ask the care nurse who will be able to give you more information.

During the post-surgery discussion in the recovery room, she may still be experiencing some effects from the anesthesia – a general anesthesia can impair understanding and memory for a few hours or even days. You can help by asking the nursing staff questions about anything that is unclear, taking notes about their advice, and reading a handout on post-lumpectomy care if it is available. Take a copy of questions she and you would like answered, outlined in Box 6.3, to make sure you don't forget anything.

After leaving the clinic or hospital, recovery time is usually short. She can probably resume normal, but not strenuous, activities within two weeks. She may appreciate social support and practical help during this recovery period from you and her family and friends.

As we recommended in the chapter on biopsies (Chapter 5) help her look out for swelling, redness, fluid buildup, fever, chills, or other signs of infection or lymphedema. With any sign of infection or other concerns, encourage her to call her doctor, quickly.

Periodic photos of the lumpectomy area, taken with a camera or cell phone, might help track her recovery and identify any adverse reactions.

Box 6.3   Questions to Ask About Her Recovery After the Lumpectomy

- How to care for the surgical site.
- How to care for the drain if she will have one at home.
- If antibiotics are prescribed, what are they?
- Will there be pain or numbness?
- Recommendations?

  - Pain relief
  - Bandaging
  - Bathing and showering
  - Exercise
  - When she may wear a bra and what types are okay
  - Diet
- What symptoms indicate that the doctor be contacted and how should they be contacted?
- What are the signs of infection?
- When will the results of the biopsy be available?
- Confirm the date of her follow-up appointment to discuss the results and future treatment recommendations.

Discomfort is usually minimal, but she may experience some mild pain, numbness, and tightness in her underarm area (see Box 6.4 for side effects of a lumpectomy). She may be given a prescription for pain medication. Often, over-the-counter medication is sufficient to relieve pain, but the doctor may recommend continuing to avoid aspirin for several days because of its increased risk of bleeding. Depending on the particular lumpectomy and recommendations from her doctor, she may be told not to resume strenuous exercise for a couple of weeks.

Results of the Lumpectomy, Follow-Up, and Recovery

Within a few days to a week or so, the pathologist will send a pathology report to her doctor. As with a biopsy, the pathologist will indicate the type of cancer found and its characteristics (e.g., invasive, noninvasive, hormone sensitivity, grade; see Boxes 2.1 and 2.3). This information is important to help the doctor discuss with her which follow-up treatment

---

Box 6.4   Possible Side Effects of a Lumpectomy

- Bleeding
- Infection
- Scar tissue formation
- Pain, tenderness, or numbness at the surgical site
- Swelling, including lymphedema which is permanent
- Stiffness
- Change in the appearance of the breast

---

would be best – another lumpectomy, a partial mastectomy, a mastectomy, radiation treatment, chemotherapy, and/or hormone therapy. The results of any genetic testing for mutations will also be a factor in deciding on subsequent treatments. She may also be given information about support groups or available behavioral health services.

More detailed information about pathology reports can be found at https://www.cancer.gov/about-cancer/diagnosis-staging/diagnosis/pathology-reports-fact-sheet#what-information-does-a-pathology-report-usually-include

Waiting for the results can be stressful. Both of you cannot help worrying about whether all the cancer was removed or if cancer was found at the edges of the tissue, which would require another surgery. Will another lumpectomy be recommended, or a mastectomy? You can be emotionally supportive and encourage her to maintain her positive social interactions, interests, and activities during this waiting period. At times of stress, research has shown it can be helpful for a person to maintain involvement in parts of their life that don't involve the source of that stress.

You can help by educating yourself about post-lumpectomy care and offer to go with her, or arrange for others to do so, during the follow-up discussions with her doctor. You or others can serve as her advocate and help clarify anything that is unclear. The goal of this appointment is to clearly understand the options for what comes next and why. It might be helpful to have a list of questions, taken from boxes in this chapter and Chapter 5. As we discuss in Chapter 3, she may also wish to explore a second medical opinion after receiving these results, an option that is generally supported by medical providers.

Exercise and Home Care

Exercise is an important part of recovery. Help her develop a good exercise routine. Join her if possible – lots of research supports the benefits of post-surgery exercise and doing it with others makes it more enjoyable for some people. Remember also that the type and amount of exercise will vary depending on the time after surgery, the effects of the surgery on arm movement, and her physical condition. Some exercises are designed to help reduce the risk of swelling in the arm on the side where the surgery occurred.

Consultation with professionals experienced with post-surgical exercises could help; in many hospitals there are Physical Therapists (PTs) who provide this service. Normal activities such as bathing, dressing, eating, and teeth and hair brushing using the arm on the side of the surgery can also be a natural way to help with recovery.

Although strenuous exercise should be avoided soon after the lumpectomy, most respected sources recommend gentle and moderate exercise beginning a few days after surgery to help her regain flexibility, movement abilities, get back to normal activities, and reduce some of the side effects of the surgery. Exercise can also improve her overall fitness, which helps in recovery.

If she is scheduled for radiation therapy after her lumpectomy, she must be able to raise her arm with her forearm flat against the side of her head; if she cannot do this, radiation will need to be postponed until she can.

Some particular exercises might be especially helpful and may be suggested by her doctor or an exercise specialist. The American Cancer Society website https://www.cancer.org/cancer/breast-cancer/treatment/surgery-for-breast-cancer/exercises-after-breast-cancer-surgery.html describes exercises that can be helpful after breast cancer surgery. This website illustrates wand, elbow winging, shoulder blade stretch and squeeze, side bends, chest wall and shoulder stretch, and other exercises. These exercises involve raising the arm above the heart, lifting the arm while lying down, hand exercises, and deep breathing. https://www.youtube.com/watch?v=CPw2Me1jUCc is a video of exercises that can be done to help regain mobility after a lumpectomy or mastectomy.

Monitoring for Potential Side Effects

The American Cancer Society (https://www.cancer.org/treatment/treatments-and-side-effects/physical-side-effects/lymphedema/for-people-with-lymphedema.html) recommends that caregivers:

1   Encourage her to watch for early signs of infection (e.g., pus, rash, red blotches, or streaks, swelling, increased heat, tenderness, chills, or fever). Taking a photo each day on your cell phone or camera might help you detect subtle changes in appearance.
2   Help make the home environment safe from possible falls.
3   Keep pets' claws trimmed to avoid scratching the patient's skin.
4   Help her avoid exposure to extreme temperatures (e.g., ice packs or heating pads).

Caring for a Surgical Drain

Some women leave the clinic with a surgical drain to help remove fluid from the breast or armpit. If she has a drain, it will usually remain until her first follow-up visit with her doctor, perhaps 1–2 weeks after surgery. At home, the fluid must be emptied through the drain bulb a few times a day. She will be instructed to measure and record the volume to determine when the drain can be removed. Most women do not need help with this fairly simple procedure, but you can assist in organizing a private space for her when she does it. Clarify with a member of her oncology team the use of a drain, its care, and when it can be removed.

Other Potential Negative Consequences of Lumpectomies

As with all surgical procedures, lumpectomies can be associated with some negative consequences. These include bleeding; infection; scar tissue formation; pain, tenderness, or numbness at the surgical site; swelling, including lymphedema (see Chapter 9 for more information about this condition) which does not subside; stiffness; and change in the appearance of the breast.

Even for small tumors, removing the cancerous tissue and a small amount of surrounding healthy tissue for testing may produce unsatisfactory cosmetic results, especially for small breast sizes. In such cases, *oncoplastic surgery* may be offered that can reshape the remaining breast tissue to approximate her pre-surgical breast appearance. Her surgical team may include a plastic surgeon in addition to an oncologist and/or breast surgeon.

Summary and Recommendations

• A lumpectomy is breast-conserving surgery involving the removal of the cancer and a small amount of healthy surrounding tissue of the breast.

- The decision about whether to do a lumpectomy or mastectomy is influenced by the characteristics of the tumor, the woman's concerns and preferences, genetics testing results, whether a previous lumpectomy has been performed followed by radiation, and other factors including her medical and family history.
- If the doctor makes a treatment recommendation, you and she should understand the basis for that decision (e.g., size, location, stage of the tumor).
- Ask about oncoplastic surgery when the amount of tissue removed (particularly in relationship to the size of her breast) could mean the cosmetic appearance of the breast is unsatisfactory after surgery.
- Be clear about how to prepare for a lumpectomy, the procedure, and follow-up care: Take a copy of Box 6.1 and takes notes about the answers to her and your questions. Assume that you are going through the procedure – what would *you* want to know.
- If she wishes, serve as her advocate and help her get information and answers to her questions.
- The lumpectomy is often performed with a general anesthetic and sometimes a local anesthetic, depending on the type of lumpectomy and the clinic that performs it.
- The tissue that was removed will be examined by a pathologist to see if there are any cancer cells left behind at the margins of the tissue.
- Most lumpectomies are performed on an outpatient basis and the woman can return home after resting for a short period in a recovery room. She will need a ride home.
- She will receive written instructions about post-surgery care. You can help by asking questions if anything is unclear, taking notes during discussions, and reading a handout on post-lumpectomy care. Take a handout of questions, outlined in Box 6.3, and ask the care nurse any questions you have before leaving.
- She may appreciate social support and practical help at home while she is recovering from the surgery.
- With any sign of infection and potential side effects, encourage her to call her doctor quickly.
- It can be stressful waiting for the biopsy results after the lumpectomy so encourage her to maintain her positive social interactions, interests, and activities while she is waiting.
- Learn about post-lumpectomy care and offer to go with her and serve as her advocate during the follow-up discussions with her doctor.
- Moderate exercise is an important part of recovery. You could help her develop a good exercise routine by doing activities together.

- A sentinel lymph node biopsy involves the removal of one or more lymph nodes into which a tumor drains (sentinel nodes) to see if the cancer has spread.

Sources for More Information

https://www.cancer.gov/about-cancer/diagnosis-staging/diagnosis/pathology-reports-fact-sheet#what-information-does-a-pathology-report-usually-include (information about pathology reports)

https://www.youtube.com/watch?v=Dp_hXw8P_7Q) (a video on deciding between a lumpectomy and mastectomy)

https://www.cancer.org/cancer/breast-cancer/treatment/surgery-for-breast-cancer/breast-conserving-surgery-lumpectomy.html (a general site with lots of links from the American Cancer Society)

https://www.cancer.org/cancer/breast-cancer/treatment/surgery-for-breast-cancer/exercises-after-breast-cancer-surgery.html (describes exercises to do after breast cancer surgery)

https://www.breastcancer.org/treatment/surgery/lumpectomy/expectations (describes what to expect before, during, and after a lumpectomy)

7 Chemotherapy

We noted in Chapter 2 that most women with breast cancer receive some form of chemotherapy either before or after surgery and in early and later stages of breast cancer. Some chemotherapy medicines are taken by mouth and others are injected into a vein or muscle, usually in a special chemotherapy room in a hospital or clinic. In some cases, chemotherapy medicines can be administered in a doctor's office and at home. We also noted that some women experience stressful side effects from chemotherapy.

In this chapter we discuss how the chemotherapy drugs work and how they are administered through ports or catheters so that you can understand what she will experience. We also discuss home injections of medicines and some of the more common side effects of chemotherapy; we emphasize how you can help her cope with likely chemotherapy procedures and their side effects.

The National Cancer Institute (NCI) offers a 60-page informative booklet on chemotherapy *"Chemotherapy and You"* https://www.cancer.gov/publications/patient-education/chemotherapy-and-you.pdf. The booklet, easily viewed on their website, discusses how chemotherapy works, how it affects cancer cells, side effects and how to manage them, and sources for additional information.

How Chemotherapy Works

There are many chemotherapy drugs and they work in different ways. However, all are designed to kill cancer cells, keep them from dividing, slow their growth, keep them from spreading within the breast or to other parts of the body, shrink cancer tumors to relieve pain, or reduce the risk of developing breast cancer or other cancers. Some of the drugs can affect cancer cells in more than one way. At the time this book was written, the NCI (https://www.cancer.gov/about-cancer/treatment/

DOI: 10.4324/9781003194088-7

drugs/breast) listed about 90 different drugs that have been approved by the Food and Drug Administration to treat breast cancer. The NCI website also lists combinations of drugs most often used. The website is useful for both patients and their supporters because once you know what drugs she will be taking, you can select that drug name on the website and you will be linked to another website that explains what it's used for, how it's used, warnings about the drug, possible side effects, how it interacts with other drugs, and ongoing clinical trials for which she may be eligible. Other medicines may also be used to control the side effects of chemotherapy drugs; to help cope with breast cancer surgery, chemotherapy, or radiation; and to help a woman keep healthy during and after treatment.

Like all cells in the body, new and immature cancer cells go through several phases of growth and development in order to become mature cancer cells. Different chemotherapy drugs target different phases of this cell growth and interrupt their typical development.

One of the negative aspects of chemotherapy is that it is a *systemic treatment* – the drugs circulate through the bloodstream and can affect many different cells in the body. The drugs are used to fight cancer because cancer cells form new cells more quickly than do other cells and the chemotherapy drugs have a stronger effect on quickly dividing cells.

Many side effects of chemotherapy occur because there are other cells in the body that also develop quickly, so chemotherapy drugs attack them as well. For example, some chemotherapy drugs attack fast growing cells in the hair (e.g., scalp, eyelids, and eyebrows), nasal cavities, intestinal track, nails, blood, and vagina. The side effects of chemotherapy vary widely, depending on the type of drug and the characteristics of the woman receiving the drug. Side effects can include fatigue, hair loss, nausea and vomiting, weight loss, low red blood cell counts, memory troubles, mouth sores, and reduced immune system functioning, among others. We discuss some of these side effects and how to help her cope with them later in this chapter.

Chemotherapy Administered Through an Implanted Port or Catheter

Chemotherapy drugs are typically administered several times across days, weeks, months, and sometimes years. Because veins can be damaged from frequent direct injections of strong drugs through the skin into the bloodstream, chemotherapy drugs for breast cancer are often delivered through an *implantable port,* or sometimes a *catheter,* attached to a vein. Receiving multiple injections through an implanted port rather than through needles repeatedly inserted into a vein is less painful and reduces damage to the vein or surrounding tissue. Those ports can also be used to draw blood or to administer other drugs.

An implantable port is a small plastic or metal disc surgically inserted just under the skin, usually close to the collar bone, on an outpatient basis. A small tube (catheter) connects the port directly to a large vein under the skin. The preparation and operating procedures for preparing for implanting the port and catheter are similar to those for a lumpectomy, described in Chapter 6 (p. 70), and may differ across hospitals and clinics. More information about the use of catheters in chemotherapy can be found at: https://www.cancer.net/navigating-cancer-care/how-cancer-treated/chemotherapy/catheters-and-ports-cancer-treatment. The video https://www.youtube.com/watch?v=VrD4E5 CAkT8 from Oregon Health Science University illustrates the placement and care of a port.

A chest X-ray may be taken after the surgery to make sure that the port and catheter are in the right place. A YouTube video (https://www.youtube.com/watch?v=JOuYz-kFXb4) from the Norton Cancer Institute explains how the port is used during chemotherapy and the care taken to prevent infection. Unless treatment is ongoing for advanced cancer, the port will be removed after the scheduled chemotherapy sessions have ended.

Helping Her with a Port or Catheter

Before the port is implanted, she will be given written instructions about how to help her care for the area. Because some chemotherapy drugs interfere with a woman's immune system and make her more susceptible to infections, it is important to properly care for her port or catheter. She should check the area around it regularly and look for signs of redness, bleeding, heat, or swelling.

She may also have to restrict her physical activity for several days after the port has been surgically implanted, and you or others may be able to help with household or other tasks during that period. She should avoid heavy lifting and strenuous exercises until the incision area has healed. After healing, she can resume normal activities, such as swimming or other exercise, and can treat the area over the port just like the rest of her skin.

Depending on the type of port and instructions from her doctor, you may also be able to help her with changing the bandage and checking that the top is clamped shut if it extends beyond the skin. She should contact her oncology team if she is experiencing any unusual symptoms,

Box 7.1   Helping Her with an Implanted Port or Catheter

- If these have not already been given to her, ask for written instructions about care for the area, how to clean the port at home if necessary, and what she may take for pain relief.
- If she would like, accompany her when she discusses the port or catheter with her doctor.
- Before the port or catheter is implanted, clarify with her doctor or surgeon what will happen during the operation, the type of anesthesia that will be used, and how she should prepare for the operation.
- Clarify instructions with her doctor or her care nurse about how to help her care for the area after the surgery and what type of pain relief she should use, if needed.
- If she has questions about whether and how to flush or clean the port at home, encourage her to ask the care nurse.
- Drive her before and after the operation.
- Help with household or other tasks for several days following the surgery and encourage her to avoid strenuous exercise for a few weeks after the surgery.
- Help her change the bandage daily.
- If you notice any signs of infection such as redness or swelling, encourage her to contact her oncology team.

such as dizziness or shortness of breath or other severe symptoms indicated in her instructions. If you and she are very concerned about any symptoms, take her to the emergency room. Box 7.1 briefly summarizes recommendations for how you can help before and after the operation.

What Happens During a Chemotherapy Session

The methods of delivering the chemotherapy drugs depend on the type of chemotherapy she receives and the clinic or hospital where she receives it. The specific procedures will be described by her doctor before the sessions start. Many chemotherapy clinics and hospitals will also have written material, educational websites, or YouTube videos that describe the chemotherapy sessions. You can help by insuring that she fully understands what will happen during a chemotherapy session to lessen any anxiety she may feel. Most chemotherapy sessions are free from discomfort, and the most frequent complaint is that they are boring.

Administration of the Chemotherapy Drugs

A well-constructed video of a typical chemotherapy session at the Ottawa Hospital in Canada can be found at https://www.youtube.com/watch?v= fzXzsdjSEaU. A longer instructional video about cancer and chemotherapy by the same hospital can be found at https://www.youtube.com/watch? v=7xJkrk-ZdLQ. Both videos show typical chemotherapy rooms, preparation for chemotherapy, the chemotherapy procedures, and discuss possible side effects of chemotherapy. Remember that her chemotherapy session may differ from that illustrated in the Ottawa Hospital videos, so clarify the procedures with her doctor before they start. Usually, once she is in the chemotherapy room, she will be seated in a comfortable recliner chair. She may be given antiemetic medicine prior to the start of a chemotherapy session to reduce nausea and vomiting side effects.

There are likely to be several other persons in the room who will also be receiving chemotherapy. The chemotherapy nurses carefully guard the privacy of other patients who are receiving chemotherapy in the same room but they may allow you to visit for a short time when she first enters the room. Sometimes, you can stay during the chemotherapy session, but this may be discouraged and often there is insufficient room. Steve visited Megumi early in her 4-hour sessions but left after about 15 minutes, and Ian also made a similar visit just to see what Luanna was going through. The nurses in the room will be wearing protective clothing to avoid contact with the chemotherapy drugs.

Beside the recliner, there may be a side table for personal items, water, and ice (she may experience a hot or dry mouth during the chemotherapy session) and sometimes a TV. She can use the time for relaxation, reading, listening to music, writing to others, catching up with friends, so may want to bring things along to keep busy. Many chemotherapy clinics also have regulations about the type of food that can be brought into the sessions (e.g., no strong smelling food) and the types of liquid containers permitted (e.g., requiring lids on drink containers).

When the medicines are ready, a nurse will prepare her port or catheter area by carefully cleaning with an antiseptic solution to reduce the chance of infections when the special needle is inserted. A pump will be attached to the port or catheter to control how much and how fast the drug goes into the vein. The administration of the chemotherapy medicine can take a few minutes or a several hours, depending on the type of medicines used and the stage of treatment. Her nurse or doctor will tell you ahead of time.

If you are unsure, ask. Video discussions and depictions of chemotherapy can be found at https://www.youtube.com/watch?v=7xJkrk-ZdLQ by Oxford University.

The Schedule of Chemotherapy

The length of time between chemotherapy sessions depends on which drugs are used and how she is responding to them. For example, some women will receive chemotherapy for several hours every two-to-four weeks. Other women may be given drugs for several days every two-three weeks. Sometimes, a drug will be administered daily at home through a catheter.

The number of days or months that drugs are injected depends on her type of cancer, the type of drugs administered during chemotherapy, and her health. Two to six months of chemotherapy is typical, but the treatments can last longer and be repeated after periodic breaks if she has advanced breast cancer.

The schedule of chemotherapy will also depend upon how the drugs affect her. This is discussed in greater detail in "**Blood Tests**" and "**Side Effects**" below. For example, if her blood tests indicate problems with her liver or kidney functioning, the next chemotherapy session might be delayed until the blood tests indicate a recovery.

Blood Tests During Chemotherapy

Two types of blood tests are routinely used during chemotherapy, usually immediately before each chemotherapy treatment, but sometimes up to 48 hours before a chemotherapy session. Their purpose is to check on her general health and to detect damage that the drugs may be causing. The blood tests can measure several effects of the chemotherapy. A *complete blood count (CBC)* is a measure of her levels of red blood cells, white blood cells, and platelets. A low white blood cell or neutrophil count indicates that she may be more susceptible to infection. Low hemoglobin indicates that she may be experiencing signs of anemia. If this is the case she may be feeling tired, fatigued, weak, or dizzy. A low blood platelet count indicates that she may be susceptible to bleeding. The *blood chemistry panel* measures the levels of chemicals, enzymes, and organic waste products that are normally found in the blood. Abnormal levels of some enzymes (alanine aminotransferase (ALT), aspartate aminotransferase (AST), alkaline phosphatase) indicate that the chemotherapy may be damaging the liver, kidney, or bone. These results may lead the oncologist to delay chemotherapy sessions for a while to allow the kidney or liver to recover (they can also indicate that the cancer has spread to the kidney or liver). She may be given medicines to take at home to reduce side effects such as infections, fatigue, and nausea.

How to Help Her with Her Chemotherapy Sessions

The chemotherapy procedure itself can be stressful and there are opportunities for you to help before, during, and after her sessions. First, offer to help and if she says that she would appreciate it, ask her how she would like you or others to help. Because people differ in the degree and kind of help they like, ask, and try to understand what she says and what she means. For example, she may be anxious, depending on what she has heard or read about receiving chemotherapy. Your support may help reduce her "anticipatory anxiety" about what will happen during and after chemotherapy sessions.

As we discuss in Chapter 3, people also differ in the way that they express their feelings and preferences. Some persons may appreciate help but be reluctant to ask for it because they do not want to inconvenience others, feel dependent, or appear weak. Some may want to feel more in control of their chemotherapy treatment or may prefer to deal with the chemotherapy process in private. Below, we list below some specific ways that you can help her before, during, and after chemotherapy:

- Before chemotherapy starts, help her clarify with her oncology team what will happen during the chemotherapy sessions. Because chemotherapy can have systemic effects, it is important that she prepare for some of those effects. It can be complicated because chemotherapy medicines differ in their side effects and women differ in their responses to chemotherapy drugs.
- Help her clarify with her doctor what side effects she could experience so that she, and you, can prepare for them. One of those effects can be an increased susceptibility to infection. https://www.breastcancer.org/treatment/chemotherapy recommends that she get a dental check-up and get her teeth cleaned to reduce the chance of infection through the mouth. A pap smear and heart test are also recommended. Additionally, some prescribed and over-the-counter medicines can interact with chemotherapy medicines. It is important that her doctor knows, before chemotherapy starts, about everything she is taking.
- You can help her clarify with her oncology team about what she should do, and not do, before she begins chemotherapy. She should be given written instructions with clear instructions about eating or

drinking before a chemotherapy session. Remember that she can be experiencing some anxiety that makes it hard for her to take in everything and remember it.

- Identify good sources of information about chemotherapy. Her hospital or clinic may offer material and we have listed others in this chapter.
- Help her keep all appointments. Regular appointments are crucial for getting better. Keep a calendar for appointments with nurses, doctors, chemotherapy sessions, blood tests, X-rays, radiation, and prescription refills.
- Help her with transportation. Many women feel fine enough to drive back and forth for chemotherapy sessions because some side effects do not occur immediately after a session. Even if she feels OK, helping her travel to and from chemotherapy sessions removes one source of stress, allows her to focus on the chemotherapy session, and provides emotional support. If she reacts negatively to the drugs or must take an intravenous injection (IV) at home, help with transportation is essential. In this case, if you cannot drive, find someone who can. Do not let her miss an appointment because of transportation problems. A taxi or other ride service is a last resort – it is not just impersonal but also exposes her to possible infections at a time when her immune system is compromised.
- Help her take care of the catheter or port. Help her regularly check her port or catheter and the area around to look for signs of infection. Depending on the type of port or catheter, you may be able to help her change the bandage, check that the top is clamped shut (if it extends beyond the skin), and flush the catheter with small amounts of saline water or sterilized water to prevent blockages in the port. Be sure to check with her doctor before doing any port care. Most ports are completely under the skin, so require minimal care. Her chemotherapy team can provide instructions on caring for the area. Be sensitive to any signs of infection and call her oncology nurse or doctor if she experiences dizziness, shortness of breath, or other unusual symptoms. Help her prepare a "chemotherapy bag." Megumi's chemotherapy bag consisted of an iPod, iPad, M&Ms, cell phone, and book. Because she may spend several hours in the chemotherapy room, this "chemo bag" will help to pass the time. The "bag" might contain food or drinks, books and magazines, cell phone, writing material, additional clothes (jacket, socks, etc. because chemotherapy rooms can be cool), tablet, laptop, reading glasses, and tissues. These are simple items that can make the chemotherapy session go more pleasantly. Because it is easy to forget

things at the last minute, you could help by making a checklist for her.
- Pick up prescribed medicines at the pharmacy during her chemotherapy session. Sometimes she will need to take home prescription and nonprescription medicines. You can pick these up for her during her chemotherapy session once they have been ordered.
- Keep yourself healthy. Breast cancer and its treatments can also be stressful for you. In Chapter 14 we discuss ways to keep yourself healthy.

Helping Her Inject Medicines at Home

Why Home Injections?

There are medicines available that her doctor might prescribe to inject at home after or between chemotherapy sessions to counteract some of the systemic effects of chemotherapy. These medicines do not directly attack cancer cells: Their main purpose is to increase the number of circulating white blood cells to help combat fatigue and nausea and to make her less susceptible to infections. If she develops infections, experiences severe nausea, or has other serious reactions, she may have to delay some of her chemotherapy sessions and thereby prolong her treatment time. An important way you can help her recover is to help her with these home injections, if she wishes.

Deciding to Give Home Injections and Learning How to Give Them

She is probably able, and may prefer, to give her own injections at home. (After each of their chemotherapy sessions, Luanna and Megumi were given a sufficient number of filgrastim syringes for one injection daily for 5 days following the chemo.) A nurse on the oncology team will show her how to do this, provide written instructions, and offer practice if she and/or you would like.

Some women find the injections less stressful if you help with them. Giving someone an injection can be an important expression of caring. If you are comfortable with giving her injections, tell her that you would like to help with the injections but ask her what she would prefer. The authors of this Guide, have had both experiences: Megumi preferred Steve to give her the injections. Ian offered, but Luanna preferred to do it herself (and found that it was far easier to do than she had anticipated).

After giving you a chance to practice, the clinic will usually supply her with prefilled syringes and give you written instructions. They may emphasize when to begin the injections (generally no sooner than 24 hours after her chemotherapy session ended), how often to give her the injections, where to give the injections, how to prepare the area for the injections, how to give the injection, and how to recognize and handle problems that might occur with the injections.

You should ensure before you leave the office or hospital that both of you are completely clear about the process and comfortable with the injection procedure. Practice in front of the nurse and ask questions if there is something you don't understand. Don't hesitate to ask someone to show you again what to do if you are uncertain. The authors have never encountered anyone on an oncology team who was unwilling to spend all the time with us that we wanted. Take notes if you feel they might help you remember how to give the injections. You could even record the procedure in the doctor's office on a smart phone or camera.

Home injections are simple to give but if you've never stuck a needle in someone or yourself, it can be stressful the first few times you do it. On the other hand, many people self-inject medications for conditions such as diabetes, so it can be done. To relax yourself and reduce the chance of errors, (1) review the written instructions provided by her oncology team or other sources of information, (2) go through the entire injection process with her, exactly as you are supposed to, but keep the cap on the needle. Practice until you feel comfortable, then you will be ready to do the real thing.

The American Cancer Society (https://www.cancer.org/treatment/treatments-and-side-effects/planning-managing/getting-treatment-at-home.html) provides guidance about home treatments, including how to inject medicines at home. Most of their suggestions are outlined below. The exact injection procedures will differ depending on the medicine being injected, but all follow the procedures outlined below.

How to Help Her with Home Injections

She will be given a supply of preloaded syringes to take home, which must be stored in a refrigerator until ready for use. It is important to take precautions to avoid an infection and to make the injections as painless as possible. We include a list of the steps involved if she would like you to help with injections. First, review all written instructions from her doctor.

1 Wash your hands thoroughly and dry them with a clean towel.
2 Ensure that she is comfortable and is wearing loose clothes at the injection site. Comfortably reclining on a couch or chair might be

best or she may prefer to stand, but make sure there is good lighting so you can both see what you are doing.

3　Prepare an area for the syringe and other supplies. There should be a convenient place to lay the syringe so that it does not touch anything after being uncapped. Place an alcohol swab, cotton swab, and partially opened Band-Aid. A new paper towel is sterile and makes an excellent surface upon which to lay your supplies.

4　Remove the preloaded syringe from the refrigerator. Allow the medicine to warm to room temperature. Usually, 30 minutes will be sufficient. Do not use hot water to warm the medicine.

5　Select the injection site. Move the injection site at least one inch for each subsequent injection. If injecting in the abdomen or belly, don't get closer than 2" from the belly button. Other common injection sites are the fleshy areas around the upper arms and buttocks, upper hip, and the top and middle areas of the thighs. Her nurse or doctor will instruct you about preferred injection sites for her.

6　Clean the injection site thoroughly with the alcohol swab and wait 10–15 seconds for it to dry. You may have to pinch her skin to make the injection but do not touch the specific injection site or blow on it.

7　Prepare the syringe – remove the protective needle cap while keeping the needle from touching anything. Grasp the body of the syringe tightly with the needle pointing up and away from you while removing the cap.

8　Check to see that the syringe contains the correct dosage.

9　If you need to place the needle down, place it on the clean area (e.g., paper towel) that you have prepared.

10　Pinch the injection site to raise the skin along with a small roll of fatty tissue – you can both do this.

11　Insert the needle quickly, smoothly, and fully at a fairly direct angle. Do not touch the plunger when inserting the needle.

12　Depress the plunger after the needle is totally inserted, gently but quickly while holding the finger grip. The best angle is usually between 45 and 90 degrees.

13　Withdraw the needle – smoothly and quickly, after the plunger has gone as far as it will go.

14　Wipe away any blood drops – with cotton swab or gauze that you placed nearby; apply a bandage if needed. There may be no bleeding or, if there is, it will stop within a few seconds.

15　Place the needle back in its protective guard if that hasn't occurred automatically.

16 Place needle in a safe container. It is recommended that used syringes be put in a sharps disposal container, which is usually supplied by your oncology team. Check with http://www.fda.gov/safesharpsdisposal for laws in your state governing the disposal of needles and syringes.
17 Wash your hands again.
18 After the injection – celebrate! You are helping her to recover and keep healthy.

Final Reminders for Helping Her with Home Injections

• Maintain a regular schedule for her injections – inject at the same time each day and follow the prescribed schedule of injections.
• If she feels unwell in any way – you or she should call her nurse or doctor immediately.

Do Not

• Give injections until you are well trained and feel comfortable.
• Remove needle cap until you are ready to use the syringe.
• Use syringe if you drop it on a hard surface – use a new one.
• Shake the prefilled syringe.
• Expose the prefilled syringe to direct sunlight.
• Keep prefilled syringe in reach of children.
• Use a syringe if the medicine is cloudy or any part of the syringe is broken or missing.
• Use a syringe if the expiration date has passed.
• Rub the injection site after the injection.
• Miss injections: If you miss one for any reason, call her nurse or doctor for instructions.

What if You Can't Be There to Help with the Injections?

It may not always be possible for you to administer the injections. If she injects herself, steps 1–18 in How to Help Her, listed above are still important. She will have to do the alcohol wiping, pinching, syringe preparation, needle insertion, and post-injection health care herself.

Do not allow an untrained person to give her an injection!

If you have been the one administering her injections, what can you do to prepare her for self-injection? Practice with her, just like you practiced before your first injection. You are now probably more comfortable with the procedures and can serve as an injection-emotional-and-informational-supportive-guide. Watch her first attempt to administer the medicine alone to see how it went – be empathic, complimentary, congratulatory, affectionate, and supportive.

Possible Side Effects from Home Injections

Medicines given at home to bolster the immune system and counter negative side effects of chemotherapy rarely have serious side effects, but any medicine can have side effects, so be observant. The most common side effects are bone pain or aches. If anything happens to her that is unusual or makes either one of you worry – call or encourage her to call her oncology nurse or doctor. We have already reviewed many signs that something might be wrong: Be sensitive to unexpected pain, headache, skin blotches, redness at injection site, dizziness, blood in urine, rash, shortness of breath, wheezing or difficulty breathing, swelling or puffiness, faintness, rapid pulse, sweating, or a general feeling of tiredness. Allergic reactions to the medicines are rare but if it occurs, take her to an emergency room.

Side Effects of Chemotherapy

We have noted earlier in this chapter that, for some women, the systemic effects of chemotherapy can have undesirable side effects ("side effects" of a chemotherapy drug are its effects other than its effects on cancer cells). The book *Cancer Caregiving A to Z* by the American Cancer Society lists 35 possible side effects of cancer treatments, most of them associated with chemotherapy. We also noted that different chemotherapy drugs have different side effects and sometimes women who take the same drug have different side effects.

Physiological side effects can include fatigue, hair loss, vomiting, weight loss, low red blood cell counts, numbness and tingling, trouble sleeping, and mouth sores, and reduced immune system functioning, among others. Chemotherapy can also have psychological effects, such as memory loss, difficulties in concentration, negative thoughts, worry, and anxiety. You may have heard the phrase "chemo brain," which refers to a temporary kind of mental cloudiness that can happen after chemotherapy sessions. We noted earlier that the National Cancer Institute website (https://www.cancer.gov/about-cancer/treatment/drugs/breast) lists possible side effects associated with about 90 different chemotherapy drugs.

Psychological and physiological side effects are often interrelated. For example, fatigue and sleep disorders can have both physiological and psychological aspects. Feeling anxious can lead to problems sleeping and poor sleep can increase a person's anxiety responses to stressful life events.

Throughout this book we incorporate research findings that both during and after treatment, breast cancer survivors can feel psychological strain associated with the diagnosis, surgery, and changes in lifestyle and social support, fear of recurrence, the physiological effects of chemotherapy, and, of course, fear of death. This Guide emphasizes how you can help her cope with this stress through social support, encouraging acceptance and optimism, and avoiding catastrophizing thoughts, in addition to the many pragmatic things you can do to help her (see Chapter 14).

In this section, we review several of the most common physiological and psychological side effects of chemotherapy and suggest ways you can help her cope with them.

Hair Loss

An early, visible, and often distressing side effect of many chemotherapy drugs is hair loss (*alopecia*). The cells and tissue that surround the hair root are particularly fast dividing, so some chemotherapy drugs will cause hair to fall out at the root. Hair on the scalp is the first to go because hair follicles on the scalp divide more quickly than hair follicles on other parts of the body.

Different chemotherapy drugs can have different effects on her hair. Some will affect mostly hair on her head; others may also affect hair in her pubic, leg, under-arm, and eyebrow areas. Some chemotherapy drugs do not affect hair growth. The hair loss may occur quickly or slowly, can lead to entire baldness, partial baldness, thinning hair, or little or no hair loss. For example, doxorubicin usually causes complete hair loss on the head during the first few weeks of treatment. Methotrexate rarely causes complete hair loss but it might thin her hair. Paclitaxe usually causes hair loss on every part of the body. Her oncology nurse or doctor can explain which side effects she should expect from the chemotherapy drugs she will be taking and she can also check https://www.cancer.gov/about-cancer/treatment/drugs/breast). This information can help her prepare, emotionally and practically, for the expected side effects, including hair loss.

Maximum loss of hair usually occurs 1–2 months after chemotherapy starts, and her scalp may feel sensitive when she is losing her hair. Megumi's hair loss started after two chemotherapy sessions, and Luanna's – already cut short as part of her advance planning – also did not begin falling out until after her second chemo session. Remind her that hair loss is a sign that the chemotherapy medicines are attacking cancer cells!

Some studies have found that cooling the scalp before, during, and after chemotherapy sessions (*scalp hypothermia*) reduces the amount of hair loss for some women. One method of cooling the scalp involves the use of *cold caps,* which are computer-controlled devices that contain a cooling fluid. The cap is placed over the head to reduce blood flow to the hair follicles, thereby reducing the amount of the chemicals that reach the hair follicles. Scalp hypothermia also reduces the activity of the hair follicles and makes them less sensitive to the chemicals. The American Cancer Society discusses the pros and cons of cold caps at https://www.cancer.org/treatment/treatments-and-side-effects/physical-side-effects/hair-loss/cold-caps.html.

Different women react differently to hair loss. Many women have commented that, despite knowing it would happen, hair loss can be shocking, anxiety-provoking, depressing, and a powerful reminder that they are not well. Empathize! Imagine yourself in her place and consider how you might feel if you have had a full head of hair and then within days it begins to fall out. She may worry about her attractiveness and what others might think about her. She looks in the mirror and sees a person who looks very different. She may not want to be seen as a cancer patient, but hair loss is a signs to everyone that she is a cancer patient. Luanna recalls that when her adult daughter and ten-year-old grandson came to spend ten days with her after her final chemotherapy session but before her surgery, she was prepared to wear her wig in the house. But, her grandson said not to worry, he knew all about cancer, and she was his grandma after all!

Some women do not mind hair loss and are not embarrassed to wear a wig or even to be seen bald in public. As noted in breast cancer.org, some women choose to go "bold and bald." As Megumi did, they use makeup and jewelry to accent their look and can appear quite fashionable. Other women are uncomfortable being seen in public without their hair and would prefer to be seen in a scarf, cap, turban, or wig.

Hair almost always grows back. Except in rare cases, her hair loss will be temporary and new hair growth can be noticed several weeks after the last chemotherapy session. In many cases, hair may start to grow back even before the chemotherapy sessions have stopped. The hair on her scalp grows more quickly and will probably start growing before hair on other parts of her body. You may notice one-inch of new hair two months after the last chemotherapy session. Her new hair may be different in terms of color, texture, or curliness and it may take a year, but her new hair will eventually be replaced by the type of hair she had prior to chemotherapy.

Box 7.2   Practical Ways to Help Her with Hair Loss

- If she has long hair, encourage her to go to a hairdresser for a short style so it will be less dramatic when she starts to lose her hair. Luanna gave up her longer hair and ended up staying with the shorter hairstyle permanently, even after her hair had returned to normal.
- *Help with Head Shaving and Trimming.* She may decide to shave her head before or during hair loss. The hair loss can be pretty spotty and clumpy at the beginning and she may prefer to have her head shaved. If you can do this skillfully and carefully, and she wants you to, shaving her head is a nice way of helping. Remember her scalp might be sensitive and she may be more prone to infections. If you are unsure of your barbering skills, find a friend or family member who might be a more skilled head shaver or use a professional barber.
- *Help With Gentle Scalp Care.* She may appreciate help with gentle shampooing. Remember that she may have some arm and shoulder mobility problems from surgery and might appreciate your help. Plus, it can be a nice and fun thing to do.
- *Help Children Understand.* As we discuss in Chapter 12, children may be upset by changes in her looks. Talk to them about the hair loss, remind them that it is temporary, make sure they know that it is an indication that the treatment is working, that she is getting better, and tell them how good she looks bald. Talking to them before the hair loss might reduce their shock at seeing a rapid change in their mother.
- *Wig/Scarf/Hat/Turban Support.* She may be interested in wigs, scarfs, turbans, or hats. She can get free wigs through the American Cancer Society and sometimes through private wig salons. Ask persons in a local cancer support group or knowledgeable persons at your cancer treatment center; oncology nurses may have lots of tips. You can help locate sources for wigs, help her pick one out, if you have any fashion sense. It may be helpful to go to a wig shop while she still has her hair so that she can match her hair color, if she desires a good match. She may be interested in selecting a new, fun hair color. One's normal hair color is usually uneven, and a wig will almost always look completely different even if the color was intended

to be the same. http://www.breastcancer.org/tips/hair_skin_
nails/wigs offers useful advice about wigs.
* *Encourage Her to Wear Sunscreen.* Her scalp will be very susceptible
to sunburn after being covered by hair all of her life. Sunscreen
or some other head covering will protect her from sunburn.

Practical Ways to Help Her Cope with Hair Loss

Remembering that women can react in many different ways to hair loss.
What can you do to help her thrive? You now know that one of your
most important tasks is to find out what would be the best way to help
and support her. Maybe you already know but if not, ask her. No matter
which types of support are best for her, let her know you care about her,
and that she is still attractive! Box 7.2 outlines several practical ways to
support her.

Anticipating an Altered Appearance

As we describe in Chapter 9, a mastectomy can also affect a woman's
body image because the appearance of her breasts can be a part of her
identity. But hair loss is visible to everyone, and the effect on her facial
appearance can also impact her self-esteem, participation in public
events, and general well-being. Women have described their hair falling
out in clumps on the pillow, sticking to their body in the shower, or
clogging up the bathtub drain. It is a visible reminder to her and others
of her illness and makes her look like a "cancer patient." Your understanding of her reaction can help you to help her cope with these
feelings.

One of the studies that reported the participants' actual self-
descriptions was conducted by Hannah Frith and her colleagues in
England with women between the ages of 35 and 68, all in heterosexual
relationships. It was common for them to report immediate anticipation
of hair loss:

> *"I just sort of sat there absolutely stunned, to think that I had to have
> chemo, and initially, and I will be honest with you, my first thought was 'oh
> my god I'm going to lose my hair."*

Some women considered their hair was one of their special features –
something that they could easily style differently and change their

appearance according to their mood or the occasion. So, be sensitive to how she sees her identity and appearance being tied to her hairstyle. Reassure her that hair loss is natural, her hair will grow back, and she might even like a completely new look.

Some women in the Frith study also reported that it made them feel better to know that they will lose their hair. One woman commented, "*I thought in my head maybe it won't happen to me, I might be lucky.*" But when she was told it was going to happen, "*then I started to come to terms with it, because I thought now I can take steps to be positive and do something about it.*" There was a great deal of discussion among the women of wanting to try out wigs and scarves and other head coverings ahead of time. Having their "camouflage" prepared made them feel ready for hair loss. Another strategy, and it would be an easy one for you as support person to suggest or encourage, was to have a much shorter haircut before chemotherapy in order to prepare partners, children, friends, and work colleagues for "the shock." Shaving their heads gave some women a greater sense of control. Women with long hair might choose to cut it short or shave it off to disguise the inevitable thinning look – shedding long hair seems to trigger especially high levels of anxiety. Shaving also promotes quicker re-growth.

This issue of "control" is a central one for your role as a support person. The "feeling of control" is a key element of psychological well-being, and it is essential that you accept and do not undermine it by assuming what she should do or feel. It is perceived control over daily emotions and the more everyday and ordinary problems that is critical. Helping her use coping strategies *before* there is a crisis, such as loss of her hair, is crucial for managing the psychological side effects of chemotherapy and other breast cancer treatments.

Fatigue

Fatigue is one of the most common effects of breast cancer and its treatments. https://www.breastcancer.org/tips/fatigue estimates that it is experienced by about 90% of breast cancer patients with cancer, and 70–80% of those who receive chemotherapy and/or radiation treatments experience moderate or severe fatigue. For those who experience fatigue, it can take many forms and the symptoms can differ across persons and time. She may feel very tired, weak, slow, heavy, run down, and exhausted, and with little energy to do the things she used to do. Physical weakness is usually an important part of fatigue.

As the National Cancer Institute (NCI) and National Comprehensive Cancer Network (NCCN) emphasize, the fatigue experienced by cancer patients is different from the fatigue that all people sometimes feel. It is more profound and unremitting. For most breast cancer patients who are experiencing fatigue, sleep and rest does not help much. Although periodic rest is important, she may feel almost as fatigued after as before she rested or slept.

While fatigue often accompanies cancer, chemotherapy, surgery, and radiation, researchers are still unclear about its causes. Probably there are many. The NCI website lists 16 possible causes of fatigue. For example, she may experience other illnesses because of lowered immune system functioning, her body uses energy to repair itself, the drugs circulating through her can directly affect her level of fatigue during treatment, and pain associated with surgeries or other treatments can also cause fatigue. She may also feel fatigued if she forces herself to be overactive; is not sleeping well; not eating well because of anemia, nausea, and taste changes; or experiences depressed mood, emotional distress, and worry about her health and cancer treatments. The important point here is that fatigue seldom occurs in isolation: It may exacerbate, and be exacerbated by, many other medical and psychological conditions.

Although she may be more quickly and thoroughly fatigued by normal exercise or exertion, cancer-related fatigue is not caused by too much exercise or exertion. As we discuss below, her symptoms of fatigue can be psychological, emotional, and cognitive, as well as physical. When fatigued, she may feel less motivated to be active in any way, have more difficulty concentrating and remembering things, and experience low mood. It could be helpful if you explored with her what she means when she says she is feeling very tired or just has no energy, or is disinclined to engage in activity that she used to enjoy.

Her fatigue may not be the same at all times. Expect to see ups and downs in her energy level and strength within and across days. She may have especially bad days or time periods within days, and she may feel more energetic and stronger on some days and parts of some days. The NCI provides a website for patients that covers many topics related to fatigue – http://www.cancer.gov/about-cancer/treatment/side-effects/fatigue/fatigue-pdq#section/_AboutThis_1.

Although some women reported that they did not feel fatigue after chemotherapy, women who did report fatigue commented that it was often greatest in the few days or week after a treatment session and begins to lessen in the subsequent week. In these cases, fatigue might also increase across the first several sessions. Fatigue can last a long time, but for many women, fatigue associated with chemotherapy and radiation begins to gradually lessen immediately after the treatments stop. But the degree and speed of recovery differs across women. Her feeling of fatigue could diminish across days, weeks, and even months.

The Wide-Ranging Impacts of Fatigue

It is easy to see how fatigue can affect all aspects of her life, and possibly yours. Her fatigue makes it difficult for her (and possibly you) to keep up with work or school and everyday chores and activities. Household activities that were simple and easy before cancer can become exhausting and challenging during and after cancer treatments, especially soon after chemotherapy sessions. Pleasurable activities that she used to engage in can become harder and less enjoyable. It may be stressful for her to engage in normal social activities with friends and family, care for and enjoy her children, interact with you, or to pursue her hobbies. She may spend more time sleeping and less time being with friends, shopping, reading, conversing with others, pursuing her hobbies, and leaving the house. Put these effects all together and it is not surprising that her sense of the quality of her life and her mood might be severely affected.

Note also how easy it is for her fatigue to affect you if you are living with her. You may also have more chores to do, less time to do the things you like to do, fewer contacts with friends and family, and fewer positive interactions with her. A natural consequence of her fatigue might be a decrease in your quality of life and mood. In Chapter 14, we also discuss ways you can stay healthy.

Cancer-related fatigue can also affect her recovery after treatment – how quickly she returns to work or school or reengages in activities she used to enjoy. In addition, it can interfere with her recovery from breast cancer. The NCI notes that if patients cannot tolerate their level of fatigue or feel that they must choose between chemotherapy and their quality of life, control of their disease may be diminished. This may be especially true in cases where the cancer is advanced. This emphasizes the importance of things you can do to help her manage her fatigue, which are discussed in "How You Can Help Her Cope with Fatigue" in the section below.

How You Can Help Her Cope with Fatigue

You may be able to help her cope with her fatigue. Things that you can do to encourage good sleep, reasonable levels of activity, and nutrition might help elevate her mood and feel less fatigued. Perhaps you want to help but are unsure how. Our recommendation repeated throughout this book: Ask her! Ask her what would be most helpful. What, when, how much, how often it would be helpful? Let her know that you are thinking about her and would like to help. The major goal for your help: Help (not push) her to be as engaged in her life as possible, even when she is feeling fatigued.

She may prefer to do some things herself even if feeling fatigued because it helps her feel more in control of her life. Being more active can also be an antidote for depression and worry. She may also appreciate help but be reluctant to ask. Megumi preferred to continue cooking and going for walks, even on days in which she felt severe fatigue because they were some of her favorite activities and lifted her spirits.

If you review the many symptoms of fatigue and the ways that it affects her life, you can already see many opportunities to help her. In helping her cope with her fatigue, you have four main goals:

1 Help her cope with her fatigue so that it doesn't interfere with her treatment.
2 Help her with tasks that she needs or wants to do.
3 Support her emotionally.
4 Help with any other aspect of her life that may worsen her fatigue.

The NCI, NCCI, and NCCN emphasize that caregivers can significantly increase the functional, emotional, and financial capacity of a patient coping with fatigue. So, your help is important to her. Below, we offer some suggestions for things you can do to help her cope with fatigue (remember to check with her about which ones she would prefer):

- Help communicate with nurses and doctors. Cancer treatments can make it difficult for her to concentrate, remember, and communicate effectively.
- Help keep track of appointments and medication schedules.
- Help her be physically active.
- Help her sleep better.
- Help her schedule and prioritize her activities.
- Encourage her to rest and to be sensitive to her level of fatigue.
- Encourage her to engage in activities that are relaxing and non-strenuous.
- Help her socialize with friends and family.

Psychological Side Effects

When people talk about the side effects of chemotherapy, they are usually referring to physiological side effects in medical terms, such as nausea, fatigue, pain, and so on, but psychological side effects are equally important, not only because they are usually distressing, but also because they can make the physiological side effects of chemotherapy worse than they might otherwise be. As a caregiver, supportive partner, or friend you can have an important influence on her psychological health during and after chemotherapy.

Negative psychological effects for women undergoing chemotherapy for breast cancer have been described many times in major research studies (e.g., Williams & Schrier (2005). The ones most often reported are anxiety, worry, having intrusive and fearful thoughts, concerns about hair loss and physical appearance, and decreased feelings of self-confidence and self-worth. It is probably evident how these psychological consequences, over a long period of time, can increase other side effects such as feelings of fatigue, sleep disturbances, and the negative impact of hair loss and other changes in appearance.

Many ideas for helping her cope with psychological side effects of chemotherapy are well-known and it is possible that the medical service that she is using will have specially trained counselors, psychologists, nurses, or psychiatrists who can offer direct clinical services, special groups, or access to videos and other helpful material. You can encourage her to make full use of these resources – they could add a valuable level of expertise to your own efforts.

Intrusive Thoughts

One psychological side effect of cancer and its treatments experienced by some women is *intrusive thoughts*. Intrusive thoughts are unwanted thoughts and images that keep coming into a person's mind. These are the sort of things that can be measured by items on a psychological questionnaire, such as *"Anything that reminds me of the experience brings back unpleasant feelings."* or *"I'm thinking about the chemotherapy when I don't want to."* If she is making comments such as these, it will be obvious to you that she is experiencing intrusive thoughts. Or, if she is not actually telling you, and when she seems to be distant or daydreaming or staring off into space, you might ask, "What's on your mind?"

Trying to suppress one's unpleasant memories or thoughts rarely makes them go away or reduces stress and anxiety associated with them. You may be able to help her reduce the stress associated with thoughts about a particularly unpleasant experience. The goal is for her to be able to recall and think about the experiences but not have a terribly distressing emotional reaction when she does. So, don't avoid discussing her experiences with cancer treatment because you think that will just upset her more. Without overtly challenging her negative comments about her experiences, and without being overly cheerful like a Mary Poppins, it may be

---

Box 7.3   Other Side Effects of Chemotherapy

- *Mouth Problems: sores, bleeding, dryness, thrush*: https:// www.mayoclinic.org/diseases-conditions/cancer/in-depth/ mouth-sores/art-20045486; https://www.macmillan.org.uk/ cancer-information-and-support/impacts-of-cancer/mouth-problems.
- *Hot flashes and night sweats*: https://www.cancer.gov/about-cancer/treatment/side-effects/hot-flashes-pdq.
- *Liver Problems*: https://www.cancer.ca/en/cancer-information/ diagnosis-and-treatment/managing-side-effects/liver-problems/? region=on.
- *Heart Problems.* https://www.breastcancer.org/treatment/ side_effects/heart_probs. https://www.cancer.net/coping-with-cancer/physical-emotional-and-social-effects-cancer/ managing-physical-side-effects/heart-problems.
- *Anemia, Low Blood Counts*: https://www.cancer.net/coping-with-cancer/physical-emotional-and-social-effects-cancer/ managing-physical-side-effects/anemia.
- *Constipation*: https://www.cancer.org/treatment/treatments-and-side-effects/physical-side-effects/stool-or-urine-changes/ constipation.html
- *Cognitive Impairment*: https://www.cancer.org/treatment/tre-atments-and-side-effects/physical-side-effects/changes-in-mood-or-thinking/chemo-brain.html.
- *Appetite Changes*: https://www.breastcancer.org/treatment/side_ effects/appetite.
- *Nausea and vomiting*: https://www.cancer.gov/about-cancer/ treatment/side-effects/nausea.

---

helpful to gently encourage discussion of these thoughts, remind her about helpful research findings, and support her when she makes positive comments about her coping and ultimate recovery.

Of course, the helpful things you could say to her will not completely eliminate all her anxieties or stop her from sometimes having recurring unhappy thoughts. However, the support you could provide, oftentimes by simply being there and figuratively (or even literally) holding her hand, can have a really beneficial effect on her anxiety levels, and yours.

Box 7.4   Ways to Help Her Feel Calmer Before or After a Chemotherapy Session

Encourage her to:

- Read, watch television, or listen to music together.
- Reminisce about pleasant times while taking a walk or looking through photos.
- Use imagination to describe yourselves in a peaceful quiet place.
- Do some simple deep breathing, muscles stretching, or relaxation exercises together, described in Chapter 14.
- Attend a support group meeting.
- Talk with her adult children, parents, or other family members, but not about breast cancer.
- Plan your next trip or vacation, starting with places she's always wanted to visit.
- Practice mindfulness by being aware of the details of your surroundings.
- Set some goals or make specific plans for the next activity she'd like to try.

Strategies to Help Her Cope with Chemotherapy

We have emphasized how to help her cope with several of the most prevalent and distressing side effects of chemotherapy – hair loss, fatigue, and psychological issues. But she may also experience other side effects. Her oncology nurse or physician may provide guidance for how to deal with these. In Box 7.3, we list other sources of help for specific side effects. These sites are directed at the cancer patient but in many cases you can help her adopt the specific recommendations.

Box 7.4 lists some additional ways you can help her feel calmer or better before and after a chemotherapy session.

Summary and Recommendations

- Chemotherapy drugs are designed to kill cancer cells, keep them from dividing or spreading, slow their growth, shrink tumors to reduce pain, or reduce the risk of developing new breast cancer.

- Chemotherapy is a systemic treatment that can affect many different cells in the body.
- Many side effects of chemotherapy occur because other cells in the body also develop quickly and chemotherapy drugs can also attack them.
- Chemotherapy drugs for breast cancer are often delivered through an implantable port, or sometimes a catheter, directly attached to a vein.
- You can help by assisting with transportation, checking the port or catheter area for signs of infection, and assisting her with daily activities after the port or catheter has been surgically implanted.
- Chemotherapy sessions can occur over days, weeks, and months and can last for hours; a personal "chemo bag" to take with her to the clinic for these sessions can help her cope and pass the time.
- Blood tests are used during chemotherapy to check on her general health and to detect damage that the drugs may be causing.
- She may have been given an anti-nausea medication, such as ondasetron, in tablet form to be taken by mouth prior to each chemotherapy session, but encourage her to ask her doctor or nurse about any further nausea symptoms should she experience these at home.
- Injections of medicines at home between chemotherapy sessions to boost the immune system reduce the chance that she will develop infections and help combat fatigue and nausea.
- With sufficient practice and her consent, you can administer home injections and/or she can administer these herself if she prefers.
- Consider how you can support her when she loses her hair which is one major side effect of chemotherapy, encouraging her to explore adaptive alternatives for the inevitable period of baldness. You can help to normalize things by increasing awareness that everyone knows about this side effect – even children – and most people are far more tolerant and accepting than we believe.
- Plan for the possibility that her chemotherapy sessions may leave her feeling fatigued for extended time periods. This may not happen to the woman you care about, but it is common enough for you to be watchful and help when you can.
- Be prepared for other side effects that may occur even after her chemotherapy sessions have been completed. Most importantly, review the written instructions from her medical team regarding symptoms that are so serious they require immediate attention and a trip to the emergency room.
- Rather than viewing her life during chemotherapy as overwhelmingly gloomy and problematic, explore strategies for both of you

to normalize your lives as much as possible and to help ensure that the cancer is not allowed to control her life and take away from her general well-being.

Sources for More Information

General Information on Cancer and Chemotherapy

American Cancer Society (2008). *Cancer Caregiving A to Z; An At-Home Guide for Patients and Families.* Atlanta, GA. American Cancer Society.
The National Cancer Institute offers a 60-page book on chemotherapy *"Chemotherapy and You"* https://www.cancer.gov/publications/patient-education/chemotherapy-and-you.pdf. The booklet, easily viewed on their website, discusses how chemotherapy works, how it affects cancer.
https://www.breastcancer.org/treatment/chemotherapy (discusses many aspects of chemotherapy)

Information on Ports and Catheters

https://www.cancer.net/navigating-cancer-care/how-cancer-treated/chemotherapy/catheters-and-ports-cancer-treatment (describes the use of catheters in chemotherapy; by *American Society of Clinical Oncology*)
https://www.breastcancer.org/treatment/chemotherapy/process/how (A description and image of a port; by Breastcancer.org)
https://www.youtube.com/watch?v=-SwAGtEYVEk (discusses chemotherapy and illustrates the use of a port (about 1:30 minutes into the 10 minute video; by UMC Health Systems)
https://www.youtube.com/watch?v=VrD4E5CAkT8 (illustrates the placement of a port; by Oregon Health Sciences University)
https://www.youtube.com/watch?v=JOuYz-kFXb4 (a video that explains the care taken to prevent infection during chemotherapy with a port; by Norton Cancer Institute)

Information on Chemotherapy Sessions

https://www.cancer.gov/about-cancer/treatment/drugs/breast (describes chemotherapy for breast cancer; National Cancer Institute)
https://www.youtube.com/watch?v=-SwAGtEYVEk (discusses chemotherapy and illustrates the use of a port (UMC Health Systems)
https://www.youtube.com/watch?v=fzXzsdjSEaU (a video of a typical chemotherapy session at the Ottawa Hospital in Canada)

https://www.youtube.com/watch?v=EiOtMbPR824 (A longer instr-uctional video about cancer and chemotherapy by Ottawa Hospital in Canada)

Information on Hair Loss

http://www.breastcancer.org/tips/hair_skin_nails/hair_loss (A series of websites on hair loss associated with chemotherapy and radiation. Briefly describes what hair loss to expect with commonly used che-motherapy medicines Adriamycin, Cytoxan, 5-fluorouracil Taxol. Separate short articles on wigs, scarves, nails, cold caps, skin care)

http://www.cancer.org/treatment/treatmentsandsideeffects/physicalsideeffe-cts/dealingwithsymptomsathome/caring-for-the-patient-with-cancer-at-home-hair-loss (American Cancer Society website that presents a little about hair loss but 13 suggestions for what she might do to cope with it (wigs, brushing, shaving, hair nets, etc.)

http://www.mayoclinic.org/tests-procedures/chemotherapy/in-depth/hair-loss/art-20046920 (A Mayo Clinic website that provides info-rmation on why chemotherapy produces hair loss, what to expect, how to cope, and radiation effects)

Information on Fatigue

https://en.wikipedia.org/wiki/Cancer-related_fatigue (provides an overview of cancer-related fatigue and additional sources of information)

https://www.cancer.gov/about-cancer/treatment/side-effects/fatigue (an overview of cancer-related fatigue and ways to cope)

Frith, H., Harcourt, D., & Fussell, A. (2007). Anticipating an altered appearance: Women undergoing chemotherapy treatment for breast cancer. *European Journal of Oncology Nursing, 11,* 385–391.

Reference

Williams, S. A., & Schrier, A. M. (2005). The role of education in managing fatigue, anxiety, and sleep disorders in women undergoing chemotherapy for breast cancer. *Applied Nursing Research, 18,* 138–147.

8 Radiation Therapy

In *radiation therapy* for breast cancer (sometimes called *radiotherapy*), beams of high energy X-rays or other particles are focused briefly on specific areas in the breast or other parts of the body, such as lymph nodes, where cancer cells have been detected or surgically removed. Unlike chemotherapy, it is a *local, targeted treatment* often given several weeks after surgery or chemotherapy and is implemented to kill any cancer cells that may have been missed during those treatments and to reduce the chance the cancer will come back. The radiation affects a cell's DNA and interferes with its ability to divide. Radiation affects all cells that are in the path of the beam but has stronger effects on cancerous cells because they are faster growing.

Radiation therapy can be used in all stages of breast cancer (see Box 2.2, p. 19) and also to treat cancer and its symptoms, such as pain, when the cancer has migrated to other parts of the body (see Chapter 13 on metastatic breast cancer). When used to treat metastatic, Stage IV breast cancer, the goals of radiation therapy are to slow the growth of the cancer and to reduce pain and bleeding. Depending upon where the cancer has metastasized, radiation therapy may be performed to open blocked airways or to lower the chances of a bone breaking.

Radiation therapy is frequently recommended after a lumpectomy (Chapter 5) to kill any remaining cancer cells: A lumpectomy followed by radiation is sometimes referred to as *breast conservation therapy*. After a lumpectomy, radiation can be directed to the whole breast (*whole-breast radiation*) or to only the part of the breast where cancer was surgically removed (*partial-breast radiation*). The latter procedure is an option especially for early-stage breast cancers or ductal carcinoma in situ (DCIS, see Box 2.1). The lymph nodes under the arm may be treated with radiation if cancer was found in one or more nodes. Sometimes, the specific area where cancer was removed may be given a "boost" of extra radiation to help prevent the cancer from returning.

DOI: 10.4324/9781003194088-8

After a mastectomy (Chapter 9), whole breast radiation can be used, or radiation can be focused on the lymph nodes to kill any remaining cancer cells. The decision on administering radiation therapy after a mastectomy will depend on: (a) whether cancer cells were found in more than one location within the breast; (b) whether cancer was also found in underarm lymph nodes; (c) the size of the tumor (large size tumors are associated with a higher rate of cancer recurrence); and (d) whether cancer cells were found in the margins of the tissue removed. The timing, sequencing, and focus of radiation therapy can be affected by plans to undergo breast reconstruction (see Chapter 10) or future plans by the woman to have (and possibly nurse) a baby. Radiation therapy can also be used to treat aggressive types of breast cancer or cancer which can't be removed with surgery.

Box 8.1 Classes and Types of Radiation Therapy

- *External radiation* (*external beam breast cancer radiation*) involves the delivery of radiation from outside the body by a large machine.
- *Hypofractionated radiation therapy* is a type of external radiation in which fewer but larger doses of radiation are aimed at the whole breast.
- *Whole breast irradiation* involves radiation treatment to the entire chest.
- *Partial-breast and accelerated partial radiation* involve radiation directed to only the part of the breast where cancer was surgically removed during a lumpectomy.
- *3D-conformal radiotherapy* is a type of accelerated partial breast irradiation in which radiation is given with special machines to aim more precisely at the tumor site.
- *Intraoperative radiation therapy* is a type of partial-breast radiation in which the radiation is delivered during breast cancer surgery.
- *Internal radiation* (*internal breast cancer radiation* or *brachytherapy*) involves the placement of radioactive cancer-killing "seeds" into the affected area through a cannula. *Interstitial brachytherapy* (using several small tubes) and *intracavitary brachytherapy* (using a small device placed during breast surgery) are two approaches to brachytherapy.

Types of Radiation Therapy

Box 8.1 describes the two main classes of radiation therapy for breast cancer: external and internal radiation *External Radiation* is the most common kind and is delivered by a large machine (a *linear accelerator*) from outside the body. *Internal Radiation* (*brachytherapy*) involves the placement of radioactive cancer-killing "seeds" into the affected area. Both classes aim radiation at the site where the cancer is, or was before being surgically removed, but internal radiation may be used after a lumpectomy but not after a mastectomy. The types of radiation therapies for breast cancer are described in https://www.cancer.org/cancer/breast-cancer/treatment/radiation-for-breast-cancer.html by the National Institutes of Health. A YouTube video at

https://www.youtube.com/watch?v=tIRAWVV6tzg by the American Society for Radiation Oncology describes the goals, methods, procedure, and side effects of breast cancer radiation therapy.

Treatment Procedures

In deciding on the dose and schedule of radiation, the radiation oncologist will consider the size of the cancer, its location, and her previous radiation treatments. Clinical trials are ongoing to investigate the optimal doses and schedule of radiation therapy for breast cancer. Her radiation oncologist can explain the latest results as they pertain to her particular type and stage of cancer.

Radiation therapy usually begins three to eight weeks after either surgery or chemotherapy has finished, whichever ended last. Before radiation therapy begins, she will meet with her radiation therapy team (see Box 2.5 p. 29). This is a good time for her to ask questions about the recommended treatment procedure and its risks and benefits. It may be helpful to go to the meeting with a list of questions take notes or record the conversation.

External Radiation

The actual external radiation treatment lasts just a few minutes, but it takes some time to prepare her for the treatment. Radiation sessions usually occur once a day, five days a week for several weeks, although treatments can vary in frequency and duration. The treatments occur at a specialized radiation clinic so travel time will also be a factor, even though the entire appointment may require only 30–60 minutes.

Her radiation oncologist might recommend *hypofractionated radiation therapy* in which fewer but larger doses of external radiation are aimed at the whole breast during daily weekday sessions. Some women receive *accelerated partial breast irradiation* in which large doses of radiation are directed only to a part of the breast and given over a shorter period of time. Sometimes, "booster sessions" are recommended to target specific high-risk areas after the regular radiation treatments have ended. Recent research has examined the risks and benefits of fewer days of larger dose treatment, and she can discuss the different treatment options and their rationale with the radiation oncologist.

Before external radiation treatments begin, measurements must be taken to ensure the radiation targets the correct location on her body and does minimal damage to surrounding tissues. To make these measurements, she will meet with her radiation team before the radiation therapy sessions begin. Often, a CT scan will be used to help locate the precise areas to be treated, so the radiation team may mark the area with an ink mark or tattoo dot to guide the radiation therapist. Computer software is used to guide the treatment location and intensity.

Upon arrival to the clinic, she will be taken to a small room to change into a gown before being escorted to the treatment room. The radiation therapist will ensure she is in the correct position on a special bed that slides into the radiation machine. The therapist leaves the room when the radiation is being delivered but can monitor and talk with her throughout the procedure. The YouTube video mentioned earlier from the American Society for Radiation Oncology, https://www.youtube.com/watch?v= tIRAWVV6tzg, illustrates these procedures.

Internal Radiation – Brachytherapy

Clinical guidelines from the American Brachytherapy Society suggest *brachytherapy* (a form of accelerated partial breast irradiation) is most appropriate for women over the age of 45 whose cancer was small, at an early stage, was removed by lumpectomy, is hormone positive, had clear margins, and with no indications of cancer in the lymph nodes. Compared with external radiation, brachytherapy delivers a larger dose of radiation over a shorter time period. It involves the placement of radioactive "seeds" around the area where the original cancer was located as this is the area with the highest likelihood of cancer recurrence. There are different types of brachytherapy (e.g. multi-catheter, balloon), so her oncology team will discuss with her and you the procedure they think is best for her.

If she is to have brachytherapy, she may leave the hospital following her lumpectomy with small, implanted tubes or catheters or a small balloon that will be used later to deliver the radiation seeds. In some cases the tubes will be surgically placed under the skin at a later time. The implanted tubes are placed in the area of the original cancer, stick out a bit, and will be stitched into place so the radioactive seeds can later be inserted. As we discussed in earlier chapters, you and she will need to be sensitive to any signs of infection.

Brachytherapy is done on an outpatient basis, but the schedule of radiation sessions is more condensed than for external radiation. In this treatment, a radioactive source is inserted by machine once or twice a day for a few minutes in the implanted radiation delivery device; the seed is removed after the treatment stops for that session. Depending on the radiation dose, treatments often occur twice daily for about five days. The seeds may be left in for 5–10 minutes and the entire session may last about an hour. In some cases, low dose internal radiation is delivered for several hours for a few days. In these cases she will remain in the hospital because the radioactive seed remains in her body for a longer time.

After the treatment is completed, the radiation cannula is removed. The area may be sore for several days or weeks afterwards. https://www.youtube.com/watch?v=Bv2gNO-iU78 by the Breast Cancer School for Patients is a YouTube video explaining the rationale and procedures of brachytherapy.

Radiation Therapy Repeated on the Same Area

A full course of radiation is usually given only once because it can permanently damage healthy skin and nearby organs such as the lungs and heart. If her oncology team recommends repeating radiation therapy on an area that was already given a full course of radiation, encourage her to inquire about the rationale, procedures, and possible side effects.

Radiation and Breast Reconstruction

Breastcancer.org notes that radiation therapy can cause complications with implant reconstruction and that a reconstructed breast may reduce the effectiveness of radiation therapy in killing cancer cells. Sometimes a tissue expander can be inserted after a mastectomy to help maintain the shape of the breast during radiation treatments and later removed and replaced by a breast implant. Of course, she and you can discuss these options with her oncology team.

Side Effects and Risks

Although both external and internal radiation sessions are painless, there can be side effects. As with chemotherapy, side effects can differ across patients who receive radiation therapy, depending on the type and location of the cancer, the type and dose of radiation, and health of the woman. Some women experience no side effects.

Early side effects can occur soon after or within weeks after radiation treatment begins, including psychological effects such as distress, anxiety, fatigue, and depression. Research suggests about 20% of breast cancer patients undergoing radiation therapy report feeling depressed and about 10% report anxiety. Up to 80% of women treated with radiation for breast cancer report acute fatigue, with chronic fatigue persisting for almost one-third of women for months and even years after treatment is concluded. While these side effects can be discouraging, they may not be so serious as to interfere with resuming most normal activities. She can, for example, safely drive herself to and from the radiation treatment sessions, although she may appreciate the company. Steve accompanied Megumi the first week of a five-day-a-week, four-week trial of external radiation therapy, but she experienced few side effects and both agreed his presence was unnecessary after that.

There can be short-term, early physical side effects associated with external radiation can include skin irritation or sensitivity, dryness, blistering, bruising, redness at the radiation site, and/or arm swelling (lymphedema). There will be no hair loss unless radiation is delivered to her scalp or other area containing hair. If hers was a partial mastectomy or lumpectomy affecting one breast only, it is safe to breast feed from the breast which was not radiated; breast feeding from a breast treated with radiation is not likely to be successful nor advisable as radiation is destructive to milk-making tissue.

Longer term or late side effects are relatively rare, but they can also be more serious. A common side effect is damage to the skin. As many as 10% of breast cancer radiation patients experience spider veins in the treated area that may appear months to years after radiation therapy has ended. These are reddish-purple veins on the surface of the skin in the breast area, across the upper part of the breast, or under the arm, caused by damage to the capillary bed. While they may fade over time, the most promising modern treatment is laser surgery.

In rare cases, radiation therapy can damage the lungs or the heart. Lung damage may occur due to increased susceptibility to bacterial infections. Although rare, lung damage can be serious and result in long-term limits to her oxygen uptake. One of Luanna's good friends who had radiation therapy following a lumpectomy experienced this: her oxygen intake in one lung was reduced to 49% initially and is not expected to recover any higher than 75%. A very small percentage of women develop heart disease, even years later. To reduce this risk, you may be able to help her reduce other heart disease risk factors such as hypertension, obesity, and smoking. Although the risk of heart disease associated with breast cancer radiation is low, her oncologist or primary care provider might recommend periodic cardiac evaluations.

Another long-term but rare side effect of radiation treatment can be the development of a secondary cancer, usually close to the site of the radiation but this can also occur at other sites. Again, the chances of this are very low and most experts consider the small risk of a new cancer is outweighed by the benefit of treating the existing cancer with radiation. Box 8.2 outlines some potential side effects of breast cancer radiation therapy. Your oncology or radiation team can tell you what side effects might occur with her specific dose, type, and schedule of radiation.

Box 8.2   Side Effects of Radiation Therapy

Early Side Effects

- Distress, anxiety, and depression
- Fatigue (see Chapter 7, p. 98 for discussion)
- Red, swollen, or sunburn-like rash on the skin where external radiation was delivered.
- Problems with breast feeding
- Breast reconstruction complications (see Chapter 10)
- Lymphedema (swelling in the arm)

Later Side Effects

- Darkening or lightening of the skin and skin atrophy (chronic radiation dermatitis)
- Spider veins on the breast, cleavage area, and/or armpit
- Additional cancers at the site of radiation therapy, such as angiosarcoma (a cancer in the lining of blood and lymph vessels), squamous cell or basal cell carcinomas (skin cancers)
- Damage to heart or lungs with whole breast radiation (rare)
- Changes in breast size, firmness, or appearance
- Damage to nerves of the arm leading to pain, numbness, or weakness in the arm, shoulder, or hand

Many of the side effects listed in Box 8.2 are rare and most disappear weeks or months after radiation therapy has stopped. Additionally, their likelihood is decreasing as radiation equipment and procedures become more sophisticated. You can both be reassured there is no residual radiation remaining in her body after treatment sessions.

Psychological Considerations

Most people have a general idea about what happens to someone during surgery and chemotherapy. In contrast, people are less likely to have an understanding of radiation therapy. When radiation therapy is recommended for your partner, loved one, friend, or relative, both her and your understanding of this might be limited and possibly scary.

Research has found that patients often have concerns about the negative effects of radiation treatments, and some studies have found breast cancer patients have more concerns about receiving radiation treatments than do other cancer patients. Common concerns reported by breast cancer patients were the possible effects of the radiation on the immune system and healthy body tissues and organs. They were also concerned it would cause pain, skin problems, fatigue, and additional cancers. Researchers have also found that after a course of radiation treatment women reported concerns with its effects on their work and home duties, mood and anxiety, concentration, memory, and about how effective it was in treating their breast cancer. Some reported that the almost daily requirement of getting to the clinic, the loss of privacy in sitting waiting with other patients, and not always seeing the same doctor, nurse, or technician each time contributed to some of the negative psychological side effects of radiation therapy. Other research has revealed fears the equipment might fail, or the dosage of radiation would be incorrect if the technician made a mistake. They also sometimes reported feeling very alone in the treatment room despite knowing the technicians were outside but close by, monitoring them through closed circuit TV. These are legitimate concerns and strengthen the importance of getting accurate information from her oncology team.

There will be many opportunities for you to help her with these concerns. First, you and she need to get as much accurate information as possible from her oncology team about what will happen during radiation treatment and its possible side effects. Encourage her to ask about any issues of concern to her. How do they know the radiation is aimed at the correct spot and how much radiation to deliver? By understanding the therapy and its possible physical and psychological side effects, you can help her better cope with the whole process. Second, you can assist her in implementing the strategies we talk about in Chapter 14 to help her manage anxiety, such as relaxation, thinking positive and pleasant thoughts, and using humor. If she wishes, discussing her concerns before and after radiation treatments might also be helpful.

How You Can Help

As we have noted in other chapters, if you are concerned about persistent and bothersome symptoms you should recommend she contact her oncology team, particularly if experiencing persistent pain, fever, or cough and unexplained lumps, swelling, and/or bruises which don't go away. Remember one of our prime recommendations: Let her know that you would like to help and ask her what would be helpful. Below, we offer some ways you could help. They are intended to help her cope with some of her concerns about and side effects of breast cancer radiation therapy, and to lessen the chance they will cause her to miss radiation therapy appointments.

One of the most important considerations during and following radiation treatment is *skin care*. Her skin will be extremely sensitive to light, touch, and pain. It may become red, swollen, irritated, blistered, or sunburned at the site of the radiation therapy. There is some evidence that good skin care can reduce risks for future serious skin problems. Her oncology or radiology teams can give her instructions for skin care, but we offer a few standard pieces of advice here: (a) she should avoid exposure to extreme heat or cold in the radiation-treated area, so she should always wash with lukewarm water; (b) she should use mild soaps and hypoallergenic laundry detergents to avoid possible skin irritants on her clothes and bed sheets; (c) she may be thankful for your help with gentle washing of her back at the area affected by the radiation.

Encourage her to ask members of her oncology team to recommend skin creams for use between radiation sessions to help moisturize her skin, reduce irritation, and provide some relief from any problem skin eruptions. She may want to forgo underarm deodorant completely during the treatment, or ask if and when it would be safe to use deodorants and which chemicals in deodorants to avoid. She should also ask for advice regarding safe sunscreen products, including for use under her swimsuit; this will continue to be a sensitive area susceptible to burns and skin damage. It's also a good time to consider wearing soft, loose fitting clothes that don't bind or irritate her skin.

She may welcome your help in shopping for soaps, laundry detergents, deodorants, clothes, and safety razors for her to use on her underarms to reduce the risk of cuts and irritation to delicate skin. As we urge in all chapters, be supportive and empathic of her as she copes and adjusts to any of the side effects she may be experiencing.

We mentioned earlier how one frequent side effect of radiation treatment can be *fatigue,* which is experienced by some women after several weeks of radiation therapy. The causes of fatigue are unclear, but it may result from damage to healthy tissue, worries about her health, or just the stress of attending daily treatment sessions week after week. Regardless of the cause, fatigue can impair the quality of her life. It is important she maintains the recommended schedule of treatment sessions and that you both ensure fatigue doesn't interfere with staying on track with appointments.

The section on *How You Can Help Her Cope with Fatigue in* Chapter 7 (p. 100) suggests many ways you can help her if she experiences fatigue. First, if she is feeling fatigued during treatment, encourage her to tell her oncology team. Remember fatigue can make it difficult to think clearly, so you may be able to help her with that communication. They can then help determine if it is a major cause of concern. We also recommended you check with her about what would be helpful when she is feeling more tired than usual. If she would appreciate this, you could help her with some of her daily living tasks around the home; help prepare for her treatment sessions; drive her to the treatment sessions; ensure both of you maintain good sleep, exercise, and eating habits; help her to relax and maintain her positive social activities; and support her communications with her radiation team about an optimum schedule for her treatments. Specific recommendations for ways to cope with the stresses of treatment are discussed in Chapter 14 and principles of communication between you and her and between her and her oncology team are discussed in Chapter 3.

Diet is another way you can help. Certain antioxidant vitamins (C, A, D, and E) should be avoided because they can diminish the effectiveness of radiation therapy to kill cancer cells. A healthy diet can help her cope with the treatments and promote their effectiveness (see Chapter 14).

Summary and Recommendations

- Radiation treatments for breast cancer focus strong X-ray beams on specific areas in the breast where cancer cells were detected and/or surgically removed; it can be used as an adjuvant treatment for all stages of breast cancer along with a lumpectomy, mastectomy, and/ or chemotherapy.
- There are several classes and types of external and internal radiation treatments.

- In external radiation, radiation is delivered by a large machine from outside the body.
- In brachytherapy, radiation is delivered through radioactive cancer-killing "seeds" placed temporarily into the affected area.
- Radiation therapy usually begins three to eight weeks after the last surgery or chemotherapy session.
- The actual radiation treatment usually lasts just a few minutes and can occur once or twice a day, five days a week, for several weeks, depending on the type of treatment and characteristics of the cancer.
- You can help her in discussions with her radiation team about the type and schedule of radiation therapy.
- A specific area is usually treated only once with a course of radiation but in some circumstances the area can be treated more than once, with special cautions.
- The effectiveness of radiation therapy may be reduced if the breast has been reconstructed.
- Radiation treatments are painless, and short- and long-term side effects can differ across patients, depending on the types of cancer and radiation treatments used.
- If you are knowledgeable about the potential psychological side effects of radiation therapy, you will be able to support her when she is experiencing distress, fatigue, anxiety, and even depression.
- Fatigue is a frequent side effect of radiation treatment, particularly after several weeks of radiation therapy.
- There are several ways you may be able to help her cope with fatigue and other short-term side effects.
- She may also experience skin problems at the radiation site. Get advice from her radiation oncologist or nurse about the kinds of skin creams she can use, and you may be able to help her select appropriate clothes, lotions, and a healthy diet.
- There can be longer-term and more serious side effects association with radiation therapy, so check her radiation therapist has provided information regarding symptoms to watch for and when these should be reported to her oncology team immediately.

Sources for More Information

https://www.breastcancer.org/treatment/radiation (an excellent site that discusses the types and timing of radiation therapy, its effects on breast reconstruction, side effects, and procedures)

https://www.youtube.com/watch?v=Bv2gNO-iU78 (a video by the Breast Cancer School for Patients that explains rationale for brachytherapy) https://www.youtube.com/watch?v=tIRAWVV6tzg (a video by the American Society for Radiation Oncology illustrating the procedures for external radiation)

Dilalla, V., Chaput, G., Williams, T., & Sultanem, K. (2020). Radiotherapy side effects: Integrating a survivorship clinical lens to better serve patients. Clinical Oncology, 27:2, 107–112. DOI: 10.3747/co.27.6233.

Murchison, S., Soo, J., Kassam, A., Ingledew, P.-A., & Hamilton, S. (2020). Breast cancer patients' perceptions of adjuvant radiotherapy: An assessment of pre-treatment knowledge and informational needs. Journal of Cancer Education, 35:4, 661–668. 10.1007/s13187-019-01507-4.

Williams, P. A., Cao, S., Yang, D., & Jennelle, R. L. (2020). Patient-reported outcomes of the relative severity of side effects from cancer radiotherapy. Supportive Care in Cancer, 28, 309–316. DOI: 10.1007/s00520-019-04820-2

9 Mastectomies

Because so much of a woman's traditional identity is sexual, maternal, and focused on her appearance, facing the prospect of a mastectomy can be devastating for a woman. From the time of puberty, her opinions about her breasts will have ranged from wishing they were different in some way to feeling confident they are right for how she sees herself – but they have been hers. No matter how professional, how intellectually oriented, how well-liked, how kind, how witty, how sporty, or how all-around terrific she is, a woman is socialized to appreciate having a nice figure – and a "nice figure" includes breasts. Her clothing tastes may be shaped by how she thinks she looks and by desires to be noticed, admired, and respected by others – both men and women. If you are her grandmother, mother, sister, adult daughter, or a woman friend helping to support her, you will know firsthand how important breasts can be. If you are her partner, husband, or wife, her breasts will mean something to you as well: they are part of the physical characteristics you associate with her. Indeed, you have never known her without breasts unless you have known one another since childhood. Her breasts are most likely an important part of your sex life together. If she has children or plans to have children, the ability to breast-feed adds yet another dimension to their importance. Later in life, she may hug her grandchildren with a full bosom: that too is part of her persona. There is nothing superficial about the dread and sadness some women feel over losing something that has been part of her for her entire adult life.

No wonder, then, choosing between a mastectomy and a breast-sparing treatment such as a lumpectomy can be complicated and fraught for many women. There are no guarantees that any treatment for breast cancer – including the complete removal of both breasts – will save her life. Yet, she is being asked to gamble away the permanent loss of one or both breasts in the hopes and on the chance that mastectomy surgery will allow her to survive. If she makes this choice, she is likely to miss her

DOI: 10.4324/9781003194088-9

breasts and occasionally wonder, in future years, if there was anything she could have done differently.

If you are her partner, whenever a mastectomy is the best possible decision to save her life, she will need to believe you love her for who she is – not for what she lost.

This chapter covers mastectomies – what they are, when they are a treatment of choice, and how they are performed. We also address how you can support a woman preparing for a mastectomy, and we discuss the risks and side effects associated with different types of mastectomies. Unlike the previous chapter focused on surgery conserving the breast, this chapter deals with situations when it is neither possible nor advisable to save one or both breasts due to the type and stage of the cancer or, less commonly, when genetic indicators place a woman at an unacceptably high risk for death from cancer. We include guidelines for recovery from mastectomy surgeries and follow-up recommendations for how you, as her support person, can help.

What Is a Mastectomy?

Unlike a breast-sparing lumpectomy, a mastectomy involves the surgical removal of all or major portions of one or both breasts. On the day before, on the morning of, or during the mastectomy surgery, one or more sentinel lymph nodes will also be removed and biopsied for the presence of cancer cells. If they test positive, most or all her underarm lymph nodes (called axillary lymph nodes) will also need to be removed, either right away or in a future surgery. If a biopsy shows the cancer has spread to lymph nodes, she may have consented to their removal at the time of the mastectomy, while she is still under general anesthesia. Alternatively, she may be given the option of deciding later, rather than waking up from surgery to find her lymph nodes have been removed – even if this choice entails an additional surgery and delay in removal of the cancer.

Box 9.1 describes the different types of mastectomies, depending upon how the surgery is done and how much breast tissue is removed.

At the time of the mastectomy, the surgical team may also perform adjuvant therapy surgeries such as a lymph node transplant and breast reconstruction. An *adjuvant therapy* is one given in addition to the primary treatment. For example, the mastectomy is the primary surgery whereas a lymph node transplant may also be done towards preventing lymphedema when all underarm lymph nodes are being removed during the mastectomy. Alternatively, adjuvant surgeries can be delayed to a future surgery after recovery from the mastectomy.

Box 9.1   Types of Mastectomies

- *Partial mastectomy*: The cancerous breast tissue is removed along with sufficient healthy nearby tissue until there are clear margins that show no cancer. In a partial mastectomy, evidence of spread involves removing a larger portion of healthy tissue along with the cancerous tissue.

- *Simple (total) mastectomy*: The entire breast is removed, including the skin, nipple, and areola along with some underarm lymph nodes. This may be recommended when more than one tumor in the breast is identified or when the risk of spread is high even if undetected.

- *Skin-sparing mastectomy*: The breast tissue, nipple, and areola are removed but most of the skin over the breast is not. There will be less scar tissue than with a simple mastectomy. Furthermore, retaining the skin makes a reconstructed breast feel more natural. This can be done when tumors are smaller and further from the skin surface of the breast.

- *Nipple-sparing mastectomy*: The breast tissue is removed, but the skin, nipple, and areola are not. This is an option for women with a small, early-stage cancer near the outer part of the breast with no cancer in the skin or near the nipple and for women with small to medium sized breasts. During surgery, the layer of breast tissue directly beneath the nipple and areola will be removed and tested for cancer cells: if cancer is present, the surgeon will then remove them as well.

- *Modified radical mastectomy*: As in a simple mastectomy, the breast is removed but lymph nodes under the arm are also removed. This axillary lymph node dissection is performed when biopsy results during surgery reveal cancer in sentinel lymph nodes.

- *Radical mastectomy*: The entire breast, axillary (underarm) lymph nodes, and the pectoral (chest wall) muscles under the breast are all removed. Once very common, this extreme surgery is now done only for large tumors growing into the pectoral muscles. Modified radical and even simple mastectomies have been shown to be just as effective with fewer negative side effects.

- *Bilateral (double) mastectomy*: Both breasts are removed. This procedure may be done even if there is evidence of cancer in only one breast when the woman is judged to be at high risk for spread of the cancer. She may have a BRCA gene mutation revealed through genetic testing or a highly aggressive cancer (e.g., triple-negative) along with a strong family history of breast cancer (see Chapter 2, p. 24). These surgeries can be nipple-sparing if testing finds no cancer in the layer directly beneath the nipple.

Risks and Side Effects

There is some evidence about the risk of local cancer recurrence with different types of breast cancer surgeries: (a) the risk for a skin-sparing mastectomy is regarded as the same as with other mastectomy types; (b) if testing reveals no cancer in or near the nipple and areola, the risk for nipple-sparing mastectomy is similar to that for other mastectomy types; and (c) the long-term survival rates for partial mastectomies and simple or bilateral mastectomies are similar for patients diagnosed with a non-aggressive, early stage cancer.

There are other risks and side effects associated with each of these types, and her doctor will be prepared to discuss these with her and you. For example, a woman may prefer to keep her nipple and areola despite possible complications. She should know there will most likely be little or no feeling in the nipple, and sexual arousal in response to touch will be absent. The nipple could end up looking out of place cosmetically. Later, if the nipple lacks adequate blood supply, it can become diseased, shrink, deformed, and even fall off. Liz O'Riordan, co-author of a recent guide to breast cancer for women (see references at the end of the chapter), describes what happened to her. After a few weeks of looking bruised, the tip became scabby and fell off – which she described as being like an infant's umbilical cord falling off – resulting in a flat nipple stump.

The woman you care about may be given a choice between mastectomy surgeries that promise to look "more normal" after surgery versus those that do not. She may want to review some of the many photos available on the web showing the results of mastectomy surgery – or she may choose not to. She does need to be aware that every type of mastectomy surgery will alter her appearance in some way. Hence, her decision involves weighing her preferences about cosmetic results against relative costs and benefits associated with each type of mastectomy. Other factors to consider will be her overall health, the type of cancer she has, the stage of her cancer, how aggressive it is, the chance of recurrence, her family history, and genetic test results where there is a strong familial history of cancer.

Helping Her Make Treatment Decisions

There will be a great deal of information for her to take on board as she makes her decision about mastectomy surgery. As her support person, you can be her sounding board and ask good questions, take good notes about what her doctors say about possible options, and be prepared to talk about the information with her after returning home. As she considers what to do, discuss both the pros and cons of each option with her – and be ready to accept her decision. She may not want to make her decision right away during the actual office visit with her doctor but will prefer to take another day or so to consider what to do. It is best not to delay decisions for too long: scheduling surgery will require additional time – and this is cancer, after all! You may have your own opinions about what is best, but this is her choice and her decision. You will need to respect her wishes. This may be one of those times to bite your tongue and keep your disagreement to yourself.

When Is a Mastectomy the Likely Treatment?

A mastectomy is likely to be the treatment of choice when her oncology team judges that breast-sparing surgery would not be successful in treating the cancer. This may be because there is a layer of cancerous tissue or more than one tumor in one or both breasts that would require multiple lumpectomies, suggesting there might be other, undetected tumors remaining after lumpectomy surgery. A mastectomy would also be prescribed for a recurrence of breast cancer after a previous lumpectomy that was followed by radiation to the breast. Another lumpectomy can be done if the previous radiation was restricted to underarm lymph nodes only, but breast tissue cannot tolerate radiation treatment a second time. As adjuvant radiation therapy often follows lumpectomies, a mastectomy may be preferable over breast-sparing surgery whenever she is unable to have radiation therapy (e.g., she may be pregnant) or does not want to risk the side effects of radiation therapy (See Chapter 8). If the woman has a connective tissue disease such as lupus or scleroderma, she may be too sensitive to the side effects to undergo radiation therapy. In cases where either a mastectomy or radiation is considered equally viable, a mastectomy may be chosen due to the difficulty of daily travel for 5–6 weeks to a radiation treatment facility that might be located far from her home.

If multiple areas of cancer are identified close together in the same breast, their removal results in a partial mastectomy (rather than a lumpectomy) because of the major change to how the breast looks after surgery. Mastectomies are also more likely to be done for inflammatory breast cancer, for tumors larger than 2 inches (5 cm), when there is evidence of cancer in one or more of her axillary lymph nodes, and for smaller tumors that are disproportionately large in relationship to her breast size. If there is a family history of breast cancer and genetic testing reveals certain mutations (e.g., a mutated BRCA gene), a mastectomy may be the preferred option for any cancer diagnosis. The association between breast cancer and BRCA gene mutations is so high that a mastectomy may even be done to prevent cancer in the future, referred to as preventive (prophylactic) or risk-reducing mastectomies.

On the other hand, if a woman's initial diagnosis of breast cancer is de novo metastatic – already advanced at Stage IV – a mastectomy is unlikely as the cancer has already spread beyond the breast.

Combinations with Other Treatments

Primary and adjuvant treatments are generally combined for maximum effectiveness. Chemotherapy is commonly prescribed as an adjuvant treatment with a mastectomy and scheduled either before or after the surgery; the sequence will depend upon the type and stage of the cancer (see also Chapter 8). Other adjuvant treatments include radiation therapy or hormone therapy. Postmastectomy regional node radiation may be recommended whenever evidence of cancer is found in the lymph nodes for more aggressive cancers but not for low-risk situations. Where the evidence of cancer spread is limited to one to two positive axillary lymph nodes, radiation is not generally advised. The toxicity of radiation therapy entails exposing the woman to additional risks, thus there should be evidence of sufficient benefit to justify that risk.

It is important to recognize that multiple treatments for cancer increase the risk for certain negative side effects following breast cancer and lymph node surgery, including lymphedema (discussed later in this chapter). You can encourage her to ask her doctors about these increased risks in relationship to the anticipated benefits in treating her cancer.

Surgery

A mastectomy is one of several treatments that may be prescribed for breast cancer, but this surgery introduces new risks as with almost any treatment. These include anesthesia effects as well as risks associated with any major invasive surgery.

General Anesthesia

A mastectomy requires general anesthesia. General anesthesia is considered safe in comparison to the risks from the surgical procedure, but several hours of general anesthesia entail additional risks. Rarely, death can occur under general anesthesia – only 1 death per 100,000 to 200,000 operations – so this will be listed along with complications as a possible negative outcome on the consent forms she signs. To manage risks, there will be an additional medical consultation with the hospital's specialist anesthesiologist prior to surgery to determine which anesthesia and relaxant drugs are safest for her, in what quantities, and in which combinations. The anesthesiologist's assessment will take basic information from forms she will complete and/or in an interview. This information will include her body mass index, medical history, allergies, previous reactions to anesthesia, age, and any additional medications she is taking. She will be asked about health-related factors including possible heart, lung, or kidney problems; excessive daily alcohol use; depression; obstructive sleep apnea; seizure disorders; high blood pressure; smoking; diabetes; and obesity.

If she has a history of drug or alcohol use, it could be dangerous to fail to disclose this to the anesthesiologist. This information can affect the amount of anesthesia in order to avoid dangerously high blood pressure or what is called *unintended intraoperative awareness*. Unintended intraoperative awareness is extremely rare, happening in only an estimated 1 in 19,000 patients. It refers to the patient being aware of the operation occurring and even feeling pain but unable to signal this because of the relaxants given with anesthesia. Her medical records will be confidential, and there is nothing to be gained by keeping secret something that could affect the outcome of major surgery and her life. Encourage her to be truthful in all the information she provides.

Surgery Preparations

She will have received detailed written instructions on how to prepare for the surgery, including not to eat or drink anything after midnight the night before surgery. If she has diabetes, a heart condition, or any other illness, she should disclose this prior to surgery so the medical team can give her specific guidance regarding any medications taken routinely.

Generally, she may take these at the usual time with a sip or two of water, but she should always ask rather than making any assumptions.

She will be cautioned to avoid taking aspirin for up to ten days before surgery along with any other blood thinning or anticoagulant medications such as warfarin that can increase bleeding (e.g., Coumadin, Jantoven). She should discontinue taking vitamin E supplements two weeks before surgery unless it is part of a multivitamin, which is considered okay. Ceasing smoking and reducing alcohol use should be top priorities for several weeks leading up to her surgery, as both have been shown to interfere with recovery. If you are also a smoker and/or consume alcohol regularly, you can be a big help by reducing your own smoking and/or alcohol consumption alongside her.

Standard practice with a mastectomy involves one overnight in the hospital following surgery, so she will likely need to prepare for this. You and she can check with her doctor when she is likely to be discharged, as some women are allowed to go home on the same day, most will have one overnight, and some may stay an extra day. Go through this list with her in the days before her surgery to remind you both of things that can be easy to forget when you are busy. Box 9.2 lists how you can help her prepare for going to the hospital.

When you arrive at the hospital, you will be able to stay with her as she checks in and until she is given a surgical gown to prepare for the surgery. You may be able to help by packing her things in the overnight bag she brought with her and later putting them in her hospital room. When it is time for the surgery, the prescribed relaxant and/or general anesthetic medications will be administered by injection, and she will be positioned on a gurney to take her to the operating room. Nursing staff will likely remain close by and check her vital signs several times prior to surgery.

As her support person, you will probably want to remain at the hospital throughout her surgery which could be as little as 90 minutes or up to several hours – especially if any adjuvant surgeries will also be done. There may be a special waiting room set aside for caregivers of surgical patients which is more comfortable than the typical, larger waiting room in a hospital for the public. Wherever you are, you could be spending hours – probably feeling anxious – not knowing anything about how the person you care about is doing; the surgeon cannot come out to talk with you until her surgery is finished. Plan for this time by bringing something along to keep yourself occupied – a good novel, a few magazines, or a well-charged tablet to play games. You may also want a snack and drinks, so it would be a good idea to have some coins and/or dollar bills for vending machines. If you choose to take a break at

Box 9.2   Preparations for Going to the Hospital for Surgery

- *Comfortable clothes*: Help her select comfortable clothing to wear to the hospital and after surgery. A two-piece loose fitting outfit or dress that zips or buttons in the front is best. Pack an overnight bag including a front-closing robe, a light sweater or shawl, and, depending on her preferences, slippers, socks, and/or flip flops.

- *Music and reading*: You could prepare a playlist with selections of her favorite music, recording it on a portable device with ear pods. Buy a few magazines for light reading in her hospital room – post-surgery is not the time for reading *War and Peace* or serious historical analyses! There may be a television in her room with a remote control, and she may prefer the ease of watching TV.

- *Personal items*: Include in her overnight bag some personal items such as a toothbrush and toothpaste, earplugs if she is comfortable wearing them (hospitals can be noisy places even in the middle of the night!), and a list of the telephone numbers of close family members and friends whom she might feel like calling.

- *Valuables*: She should not wear jewelry or take any valuable items with her such as her purse, credit cards, documents, cash, a tablet, or any other item she would not want to lose. Hospital staff are watching over her – not her belongings – and hospitals are busy places with people coming and going at all hours. She may have her cellphone, and you could offer to keep it while she is in surgery then pass it onto her once she is awake in her hospital room. You can be a big help by holding onto anything else she would like to have during your visits (e.g., her purse). This should work for her, as you are likely to be there much of the time unless she is sleeping, in the toilet, or busy with her doctors.

- *Reporting for surgery on the day*: She may want to drive to the hospital, but you, or someone else, will be driving her home as she should not drive for at least 2–4 weeks after her surgery. She must arrive several hours in advance of her scheduled surgery, so you will be able to sit with her and talk prior to the operation.

- *Contact with family and friends*: Tell close family members and friends they may contact you – not her directly – before, during, and after the surgery as their first port-of-call. Discourage them from calling her cellphone or the hospital room phone directly; they will have no way of knowing if she is available, sleeping, in the middle of a medical consultation, or in the bathroom when they call. She may be having a much-needed nap; she may have a roommate also recovering from surgery who would not appreciate random cellphone calls. Ask callers to use your number to contact you first to check if she is available. If she is awake and up to it, you can pass the phone over to her to talk or she may set a time to call close family members and friends herself. If she does not have a contact list in her cellphone, take out that list of phone numbers you prepared for her and put it in the drawer on her nightstand next to her hospital bed.
- *Medications*: She should check with her doctor regarding taking any prescription and nonprescription medications before surgery and when these can be resumed after surgery. If her doctor says this is okay, include scheduled dosages of any prescription medications in her overnight bag to cover the time she is in the hospital.

the hospital cafeteria or a nearby coffee shop, make sure the relevant staff attendant knows how to reach you if needed and when she is out of surgery.

After the surgery, she will be transferred to a recovery room where she will stay until fully conscious. This could take another 45 minutes to an hour or so. As her support person, you may be admitted to this recovery room after her surgery, and there may even be a chair for you to sit at her side as she awakens. If you know she was concerned about some aspect before the surgery, try to have an answer for her should she wake up asking about this. The first thing Luanna wanted to know right away in the recovery room was whether her lymph nodes revealed cancer and had to be removed. Knowing the answer to this question was reassuring, and she would have wanted to know the answer either way – rather than lying there worrying.

The anesthesiologist will check on her before releasing her from the recovery room to her hospital room: she may be groggy for a few hours afterwards and is likely to be medicated intravenously for pain relief. Once back in her hospital room, a nurse will tell her the schedule for drip-feeding that medication and how she will be able – within limits – to add an extra amount of this medication herself if the pain increases. Be sure you and she know how to do this and how to summon a nurse for assistance if needed.

Wound and Drain Care at Home

You and she will be given detailed instructions in writing on how to care for her surgery site. Read through these instructions with her before her surgeon checks on her after the operation before discharge. If either of you have questions about anything in the instructions, ask her doctor at that final check-up before she leaves the hospital. Be sure you have her written copy of what to do before you leave the hospital. If anything on the list is still unclear, ask the nurse looking after her to explain procedures to both of you – and even show you what to do.

The written instructions will include specific information about her drain for a simple mastectomy or drains if she has had a bilateral mastectomy. Each drain will be a plastic or rubber tube coming out of the surgery site – usually where there are stitches which help hold it in place – to allow fluid that collects during healing to drain from the body. There will be a flexible bulb-like container at the end of the tube which must be emptied regularly, recording the volume of fluid. This record is important to monitor how much fluid is being drained, which determines when the drain/s can be removed. The tube may be long enough to place on a counter, but most likely will require her to wear a lanyard (or two, for two drains) holding the fluid-filling bulb so that it is not hanging from and pulling on her incision. One of the things you can help her with is finding a lanyard she can wear under her clothes. You may also be able to find an adapted post-surgical bra with pouches at the sides to hold the drain bulbs. She will probably not want to go out in public with the tube and bulb visible to others during the week or two while the drains are still in place.

After the surgery, she will need a private space in a bathroom so she can empty the drains into the small measuring cup the hospital will provide. She must also monitor and record the color of the fluid from her body, which should progress from a red color initially to a yellow-red and then a straw color near the time when the drains can be removed. She will need to empty her drains every few hours at first, then less often after the first couple of days, measuring and keeping a record of the volume of fluid per unit of time. When the amount of fluid reduces to the prescribed level indicated in the written instructions, the drain will be removed at the hospital during a visit. Typically, in a bilateral mastectomy, one drain can be removed several days before the second one. The awkwardness of these drains and her need for some privacy will require your support for at least a week or two, and possibly longer: Luanna's first drain wasn't removed until 10 days after the surgery and the second after another 5 days.

There are many YouTube videos that demonstrate how to care for a "mastectomy drain." Most are produced by hospitals or clinics to inform their mastectomy patients about how to care for their particular type of drain, so your procedures might be different. One good example is https://www.youtube.com/watch?v=eNCay6pkYb0 produced by Alberta Health Services in Canada. Written instructions along with a video produced by Memorial Sloan Kettering Cancer Center can be found at https://www.mskcc.org/cancer-care/patient-education/caring-your-jackson-pratt-drain.

Side Effects and Complications

The side effects of mastectomy surgery depend on the type of mastectomy, so the more extensive the surgery the more likely there may be side effects. The written instructions she received at the hospital prior to discharge will have specific information about how to cope, but encourage her to contact her nurse or doctor right away for symptoms such as the following:

- *A negative reaction to anesthesia* – her instructions will tell you what to watch for.
- *Pain, a feeling of intense pressure, or tenderness that is not improving after a few days.*
- *Swelling at or near the site of surgery.* Some swelling or lumpiness around the wound edges is normal and should flatten in 6–8 weeks. Do not use hot or cold packs near or on the wound.
- *A hematoma,* which is a buildup of blood in the wound. Some post-surgery bruising is normal and will disappear in 2–3 weeks. Treatment may be needed for bruising resulting from a hematoma: the bandage compression is designed to help prevent this.
- *A seroma,* which is a buildup of clear fluid in the wound. Again, the bandage compression will help prevent this, and the drains allow excess fluid to flow away from the wound. If the swelling does not decrease within a month, her doctor may need to use a needle to drain the area.
- *Fluid in the drain/s remains cherry red or yellow-red and does not change to a straw color within a few days.*

- *Restricted arm and/or shoulder movement that doesn't seem to be improving over time.*
- *Numbness in the chest or upper arm, beyond the initial and normal tingling or numbness on the inner part of your upper arm or in your armpit.*
- *Nerve pain in the chest wall, armpit, and/or arm that continues long after surgery.* This is called post-mastectomy pain syndrome, PMPS.
- *Bleeding or infection at the surgery site*: watch for redness or swelling of the incision, blood oozing from the wound, and/or pus or a foul-smelling drainage. She may also have a fever.
- *Delayed wound healing*: a small area of skin may wither and require trimming by her surgeon. This does not happen often and is not considered a serious complication.
- *Lymphedema* may develop after removal of the axillary lymph nodes (see the next section for more detail).

Some of these symptoms will require medical attention including additional pain medications, antibiotics, and possibly follow-up surgery, which could be minor.

If your surgery has also included the initial steps of breast reconstruction (such as placement of an expander) at the same time as the mastectomy, other problems that can occur include:

- *Poor healing*
- *A leak or tear of your breast expander or implant*
- *Scar tissue around the expander or implant*

We cover more information regarding breast reconstruction surgery in Chapter 10.

Lymphedema

As noted in Chapter 6, the lymphatic system is an important vascular system that performs multiple essential functions in the body, including immune control. The network of lymphatic vessels and lymph nodes located throughout the body transport fluid, immune cells, and other carriers important for blood plasma and other bodily functions. When breast cancer spreads, it first appears in nearby lymph nodes under the arm, near the collarbone, or near the breastbone. Because lymph nodes transport fluids throughout the body, they become the major transporter of cancer cells to other locations and organs.

When the cancer has spread to underarm lymph nodes, these nodes must be removed. If no axillary lymph nodes are left to drain fluid in the underarm area, the woman is at risk for a condition called lymphedema after a mastectomy. The risk increases when her treatment also includes chemotherapy, radiation, and/or hormonal therapy: In 2020, the risk for developing lymphedema was 1 in 3 for women who underwent combinations of therapies for breast cancer.

Lymphedema causes a permanent swelling of the arms and hands resulting from excess fluid which is not being drained. Technically, it is caused by a blockage of the lymphatic system. Early symptoms of lymphedema that should send her to her doctor right away include:

• Swelling of the arm, hand, and/or fingers
• A sensation of heaviness or tightness in the arm
• Restricted range of motion, such as not being able to reach very far
• Aching and discomfort in the arm
• Persistent infections from small cuts on the arm, hand, or finger
• Fibrosis, which is a hardening and thickening of the skin.

If lymphedema results from lymph node surgery, the swelling could be scarcely noticeable, or it could be so extreme that it is difficult to move the arm or hand. Lymphedema does not necessarily happen right away after the surgery: it can develop months or even years later.

There is no cure, but there are things a woman can do to reduce swelling and help to control the pain and discomfort. These are also things you could help her with and encourage her to do:

• *Exercise* – movement of the arm encourages fluid drainage and helps make everyday tasks easier. These exercises should not be strenuous but require only gentle muscle use in the arm and hand. You can find guidance for her regarding these exercises at https://www.breastcancer.org/treatment/lymphedema/exercise.
• *Wraps* – compression bandages discourage fluid buildup in the hand and arm, wrapped tightest around the fingers, then the hand, and wrapped more loosely as the bandage goes further up the arm. She will need you to do this for her, letting you know how tight each section feels as you go.
• *Massage* – there are special massage techniques to encourage the flow of fluid out of the arm but be sure her massage therapist is trained in these techniques. You could help with the massages, but first you need to be trained in their safe practice.
• *Compression garments and devices* – these are recommended during exercise and doing chores. She may need your help putting them on and taking them off.

- *Surgery* – in extreme cases, surgery may be recommended to remove excess tissue and reduce swelling.

Her healthcare services may also include access to specialized surgical treatment options such as vascularized lymph node transfer surgery (or lymphovenous transplant) or lymphaticovenular bypass (or anastomosis). Both these surgical procedures have been shown to improve lymphedema symptoms, but the latter is only possible when there are some lymphatic vessels remaining.

There are now options available to combine mastectomy surgery with lymphatic surgery for optimum outcomes. If her underarm lymph nodes reveal cancer and must be removed, a lymph node transplant might be performed while she is still under general anesthesia. This transplant could also be performed later to relieve negative symptoms even after lymphedema has developed. A lymph node transplant involves taking a piece of tissue with cancer-free lymph nodes, lymphatic vessels, and the small blood vessels carrying blood to tissue from another part of her body, such as the groin. The donor lymph nodes would be transplanted to her underarm/s, and a plastic surgeon will perform microscopic surgery to connect the new blood vessels to blood vessels in her underarm. Following surgery, the lymphatic vessels "take root" and become capable of moving excess fluid away from the arm, hand, and fingers in the normal way through her blood vessels, relieving or even preventing future swelling.

You can find more information about treatments for lymphedema at specialized clinics such as the Mayo Clinic and Johns Hopkins Medicine – see, for example: https://www.hopkinsmedicine.org/plastic_reconstructive_surgery/services-appts/lymphedema.html.

Recovery from a Mastectomy

A mastectomy is a surgical procedure involving major tissue injury. There are other surgeries known to be more painful than mastectomies, but do not underestimate what she is going through. Luanna lightheartedly described the aftermath of a double mastectomy as what it must feel like after a truck has run over your chest – not pleasant by any means. To combat the pain and/or feeling of pressure, the woman you care about may be prescribed painkillers right after her mastectomy, then advised to shift to an over-the-counter drug such as paracetamol and anti-inflammatory drugs. Most women report being uncomfortable for weeks or even months afterwards.

One of her biggest challenges will be sleeping at night after the mastectomy. She may have to sleep partially sitting up for a few days, as it may be too uncomfortable sleeping flat on her back at first. She may have to sleep partially upright and then on her back for up to two weeks. She cannot sleep on her side until at least two weeks and on her stomach for at least four weeks after surgery. Unless she typically sleeps on her back this may require getting used to! Cindy Boss describes how the aching and tenderness made it impossible for her to sleep comfortably in her bed, forcing her to sleep upright on a couch for about three weeks (see Sources for More Information at the end of this chapter). Box 9.3 includes some suggestions to prepare for and organize sleeping arrangements for her during this initial healing period.

Most women will begin to feel normal and resume all their usual activities within a month. Her recovery time may be longer when reconstruction is also begun during the mastectomy and involves artificial implants at the time of the mastectomy or inserting an expander that will be swapped over to a more permanent implant later. If her breast reconstruction involves tissue flap surgical procedures, her recovery time will be considerably longer (see Chapter 10).

General anesthesia also produces after-effects. Conventional wisdom is that for every hour under general anesthesia, she will feel fatigued for a full day. Most people are back to normal mentally within 24 hours, even though the medications are not eliminated from the body for up to a week. If her surgery took several hours, she may feel tired for several days – just from the anesthesia. In addition to drowsiness, she may experience slower reaction times, difficulty concentrating and remembering new information, and find complex tasks challenging. These after-effects should wear off over time.

There are steps both of you can take to prevent side effects and aid her recovery. Continue avoiding smoking and alcohol use at least until her wounds are healed. Movement and activity are good for her, so offering to get back to a daily walk together would be helpful. She may experience swelling in her arm on the side where the surgery was done. Help her organize pillows to raise her arm while she is sitting on the sofa or in a chair watching TV or reading.

You can also help speed up her recovery by helping her get to sleep. Avoid stimulants such as caffeine prior to bedtime, which should be at a regular time every night. You could dim the lights for her and encourage her to engage in restful activities such as reading an hour or so before going to sleep. If you and she prefer watching television before bedtime, choose carefully to avoid programs likely to arouse strong emotions like anxiety or fear.

Box 9.3   Coming Home from the Hospital

- *Hospital instructions*: Make an extra copy of the written instructions given to your partner at discharge so you will have one copy for her and one for you. Read these carefully so you know what is expected.

- *Sleeping arrangements*: If you can, make up the bed in a spare room for one of you to use for the first two weeks after she comes home; you will both sleep better in separate beds, and you both need your sleep at this time. If you have a recliner, she may want to train herself to sleep in the recliner for a few days prior to surgery and may even choose to sleep there until her drains are removed. If you haven't got a recliner, a bed-lounge reading pillow or backrest pillow (available at your local discount store or online) and propped up with extra pillows at her lower back may help her sleep in a partially reclining position.

- *Bathroom privacy*: Locate space in a bathroom close to where she is sleeping at night and clear a space for her to have what she needs for drain care and keeping a record of the amount of fluid. If you can, organize a small, open plastic box just large enough to hold the measuring container, the record sheet, and a pen. She will feel better if she can put these materials somewhere private but within easy reach when she needs them. It will not be comfortable for her to bend down to retrieve things from a low cupboard, for example.

- *Post-surgery bandaging*: She is likely to come home from the hospital with a post-op bandage dressing covered by a compression breast wrap around her chest to help reduce bruising, swelling, and incidences of hematomas following surgery. The wrap will be fixed with Velcro so she can adjust it for comfort; she might want it slightly looser for sleeping at night, for example. Her dressing will be removed at a follow-up appointment in 7–10 days, and her sutures will also be removed in 1–2 weeks (there may also be self-absorbing sutures you cannot see). When this happens will depend upon how well her wound is healing and when the drains are removed. As we discussed in Side Effects and Complications earlier, her written instructions will tell her what to do if she suspects something is wrong with the incision. Before you leave the hospital, remember to talk with the nurse about care for her dressing and what to do if anything seems amiss.

- *Bathing and showering:* The dressing must be kept completely dry for 48 hours so she cannot bathe or shower during that time – a sponge bath will have to do. After those first two days home, she can bathe or shower again but must try to keep the bandage over her chest area as dry as possible. Some recommend waiting at least a week after surgery before taking a shower. This may sound silly, but Ian helped Luanna wrap the post-surgery bandaging with saran wrap around her chest for showering to keep the water out – removing the saran wrap after drying with a towel. It worked!

- *Post-mastectomy wraps and supports:* Once the dressing is removed, she will be in the mood for a more comfortable and nicer-looking bra arrangement. While she still has one or two drains, she will need a lanyard to hold them in place. If you can afford something she might use for only 2–3 weeks, you can purchase what is called a "management bra" made of machine washable, comfortable fabric with hook-and-eye or Velcro closures at the front and on the shoulder to make it easier for her to put it on and remove it. Some even include side-opening for the drain tubes and pouches for the fluid containers, positioned at the waist close to her sides.

- *Post-mastectomy bras and prostheses:* She should check on recommendations for the correct bra she can wear after surgery, depending on her procedure. Some surgeons recommend against wearing a bra for some time after tissue flap breast reconstruction because they cause pressure. Later, she will need a special bra that provides good support (but no underwires), is made of soft fabric, has front-adjustable straps and closures, and a wide band under the breast area for comfort. If she is not undergoing breast reconstruction but plans to wear prostheses, she will need a bra with pockets. Most lingerie sections of department or discount stores will have suitable bras, and you can find an almost unlimited number of different options online. *Encourage her to ask her nurse when it is okay to begin wearing a bra again, what type of bra is recommended, and to get advice about what prostheses she can purchase to use.*

- *Skin care:* Her skin may be bruised right after surgery, but the bruises will disappear after a few days. Be sure she has safety razors and a wall mirror for underarm shaving to avoid irritating the incision area. As her incision heals, the scar tissue that is forming will feel thick and hard, so shop for a mild lotion, vitamin E oil, or pure lanoline for her to massage into the area *after the incision is healed, of course.* The incision should soften after several weeks, but she should avoid using any product containing alcohol or highly perfumed soaps, shampoos, and lotions.

- *Pain relief*: She will be given a prescription for pain management after returning home. Some pain killers can cause constipation, so she should drink plenty of fluids and may even need a mild laxative or stool softener. Ask if she can also take an over-the-counter pain reliever in addition to or even instead of this stronger medication if she wishes. She should not take aspirin or products with aspirin for up to 10 days prior to and several days after surgery, as aspirin is a blood thinner and interferes with clotting.

- *Post-surgery exercise and activity*: You can help by checking with her doctor about what kind of exercise is safe and when she can begin something like a daily stretching exercise to regain mobility. If adjuvant therapy includes radiation, it is crucial she can raise both arms above her head with her forearms against her ears, or radiation would have to be delayed until she can do this. She can begin to do this gradually after a week or two with useful exercises such as arm lifts, arm swings, and "wall climbing." You can find instructions on the web for her and show these to the nurse to get advice about when she can start these. She should not drive until after her drains are removed.

- *Clothing*: She will need several comfortable blouses that fasten at the front as well as comfortable pajamas she can easily put on despite restricted range of motion for a few weeks. These will also need to be loose enough to accommodate the drain paraphernalia for from 1 to 3 weeks. Our advice is to shop at a low-cost discount store or second-hand store and to spend as little as possible on these clothing items: Luanna never wanted to wear any of them ever again once she was fully recovered!

- *Physical affection and touch*: If you are her husband, wife, or partner – or even a close family member or friend – you will want to reassure her you care by wanting to hug her. Close physical contact with her upper body and especially her chest – as in a hug – is likely to be very uncomfortable for perhaps weeks after her surgery. During the COVID pandemic, most of us learned to substitute elbow and fist bumps with handshakes, and now is the time to find a hug-alternative for at least a few weeks until her chest is healed. Talk with her about how you can express affection in ways that will not hurt. Tell your children and others what to do: Touching cheeks while lightly placing one's hands on her shoulders – but keeping at least a few inches away from her body – can be just as affectionate as a tight hug and does not risk pain or discomfort!

Box 9.3 is focused on preparations for returning home after the surgery. She is going to need your help both to organize things for her return and create comfortable spaces for after-surgery tasks and care. Your circumstances and preferences will dictate if and how you can make the kinds of arrangements we suggest in Box 9.3. But there are many things you can do to help, some of which should be set up before she leaves home for the surgery. Remember, she will be feeling weak and unable to move comfortably for some days after surgery, so she will need your support.

Follow-Up

If her mastectomy included breast reconstruction, she will be scheduled for regular follow-up visits to complete this process (see Chapter 10). Following a simple or bilateral mastectomy without breast reconstruction, her follow-up schedule with her oncology team will vary based on the type of breast cancer she has, how advanced it was when detected, and whether additional treatments are planned. Typically, there will be at least one follow-up office visit with her surgeon, who is likely to be different from the oncologist who is her primary physician contact throughout her cancer treatment. Her oncologist will schedule office examination visits for her once every six months at first and less often after the first few years if there are no symptoms of a recurrence. After five years, these appointments are likely to be annual.

If she has had a simple mastectomy, she should schedule a mammogram on her remaining breast annually. If she is taking a hormone drug (such as tamoxifen or toremifene as an adjuvant treatment) and she still has her uterus, she needs an annual pelvic exam because of the increased risk of uterine cancer – highest in women past menopause. She should be on the lookout for any vaginal bleeding or spotting after menopause or between periods as this can be a sign of uterine cancer.

A hormone drug called an aromatase inhibitor for early-stage breast cancer can also affect bone density, so her doctor may set up a schedule to monitor or test her bone density periodically.

Whenever any symptoms occur suggesting a recurrence of the cancer or a new cancer following a mastectomy, other tests may be prescribed including X-ray, CT scan, PET scan, MRI scan, bone scan, and/or a biopsy.

Keeping track of her cancer treatment information can be a big job. You can help by keeping a "cancer diary" and even setting up a filing system with organizational headings for important information such as mammogram results, information on diagnoses, different treatment records, and recommendations of the timing for future appointments. Your health care provider may offer a template *survivorship care plan* for follow-up, other tests needed in the future, possible late- or long-term side effects from your treatment, and signs of recurrence to watch for. These plans typically also include suggestions for a healthy diet, exercise, and lifestyle modifications as well (see also Chapter 2, pp. 28–31). The American Cancer Society has a helpful website for follow-up care after breast cancer treatment at https://www.cancer.org

Summary and Recommendations

- Do not underestimate the value of her breasts to the woman you care about. From puberty, they may have been core to her sexual, maternal, and/or feminine identity. Even if she feels her breasts are not all that important, the permanent loss of one or both breasts is unlikely to be easy for her.
- The choice between breast-sparing surgery and a mastectomy will depend on factors such as her type of cancer, the stage of her cancer, her overall health condition, the presence of genetic mutations, and her familial history of breast cancer.
- Mastectomy surgery is often accompanied by adjuvant therapies such as chemotherapy, radiation, and/or hormonal therapy. Each of these adds to the increased benefit but also increased side effects, including additional risks for developing a complication such as lymphedema.
- Pre-surgery written instructions from the oncology team and her hospital will be crucial for you to be able to help her prepare for the surgery and hospital stay. Always read these through carefully at least three times – right away when they are given to you (asking questions if you don't understand something), later at home after

you both have had time to review what you have been told and think about things, and then again at least a day before she reports to the hospital for her surgery.

- Post-surgery written instructions are equally important so you can support her after she returns home with her daily activities and the care of her surgical wounds and drains. Again, read these together at least three times – right away when they are given to you (asking questions if you don't understand something), later at home after she has been discharged from the hospital, and then again at about the time her drains are removed. There will be things you missed earlier!

- In addition to the medical advice given to her about care after-surgery care, discuss with her the kinds of arrangements at home and other preparations you can make so she is as comfortable as possible in the weeks after she comes home from the hospital. *Don't hesitate to ask others – her mom, her sister, a close friend, her children – if there is something in particular that they can do to help.*

- Learn as much as you can about the symptoms and signs of side effects, encouraging her to seek medical advice when something seems amiss. *Don't wait!* Her doctors are there for her and would prefer to know right away when something needs attention – not days later when things are likely to be more complicated.

- Talk together about how to express physical affection after her mastectomy to avoid what could otherwise be inevitable tight hugs – that can cause her pain and discomfort – from well-meaning and loving people in her life, including you and her children. Don't "forbid" expressions of love but instead come up with good ideas about alternatives such as touching cheeks.

- Help her schedule and keep regular follow-up appointments with her breast surgeon, the oncologist, and, if reconstruction was part of her surgery, the plastic surgeon. As you have already done for previous appointments and consultations, be her note-taker and sounding-board for questions and concerns. Agree with her in advance of appointments about questions to ask and offer to participate in the conversation with her medical team if she would like.

- Check if her health care provider or oncology team offers a survivorship care plan template that you and she can tailor for your needs and preferences. You can use the ASCO template available for personal use if your provider does not already have one for you.

Sources for More Information

https://www.medicalnewstoday.com/articles/322760 (a general discussion of the stages and treatments for breast cancer)

https://www.cancer.org/cancer/breast-cancer/treatment/surgery-for-breast-cancer/mastectomy.html (a discussion of mastectomies by the American Cancer Society)

https://www.breastcancer.org/treatment/surgery/mastectomy (a discussion of mastectomies)

Aldrich, M. B., Rasmussen, J. C., Fife, C. E., Shaitelman, S. F., & Sevick-Muraca, E. M. (2020). The development and treatment of lymphatic dysfunction in cancer patients and survivors. Cancers (Basel), 12:8, 2280. 10.3390/cancers12082280

Boss, C., & Boss, C. (2017). I have cancer, now what? 12 things you, your spouse, and your family must know in your battle with cancer. Sanger, CA: Familius (www.familius.com)

Greenhalgh, T., & O'Riordan, L. (2018). The complete guide to breast cancer: How to feel empowered and take control. London: Vermilion.

Helms, R. L., O'Hea, E. L., & Corso, M. (2008). Body image issues in women with breast cancer. Psychology, Health and Medicine, 13:3, 313–325. 10.1080/13548500701405509

10 Breast Reconstruction

For a woman, a mastectomy means the loss of all or a major part of one or both breasts. No matter how she regards her breasts prior to a breast cancer diagnosis, the mastectomy can be a major blow in her life. Her decisions about breast reconstruction surgery may be as challenging for her as her cancer treatment decisions.

Breast reconstruction is not life saving, as mastectomies can be. She may choose to "go flat," as do more than half of women in the U.S. after mastectomy surgery. There can be many good reasons why some women do not care about reconstruction. For other women, breast reconstruction can help her adjust to a changed body. Different options are available that can create the appearance of the breasts she lost due to cancer.

Many aspects of preparing for breast reconstruction surgery and advice after leaving the hospital will be virtually identical to those described in Chapter 9 for mastectomy surgery, hence we sometimes refer you to material in that chapter.

Choosing "Going Flat" or Breast Reconstruction

Recent figures in the U.S. reveal that more than half of women chose what is referred to as "going flat" after mastectomy surgery rather than undergoing breast reconstruction. For a woman who chooses going flat, the mastectomy to remove her breasts generally results in a long scar from below the armpit to the center of her chest, which will be flat after the surgery. There can be various reasons for this choice. Going flat means a shorter post-surgery recovery time, less pain and risk, and lower expenses including the time otherwise lost during treatment and recovery for more complicated reconstruction surgeries. She may have other medical risk factors such as diabetes or heart problems that make going flat smarter for her. In addition, some women have no interest in reconstruction, viewing the loss of breasts as unimportant and/or having

DOI: 10.4324/9781003194088-10

little to do with their identity. Removing an implant and going flat may also be the best choice after an unsatisfactory breast reconstruction or complications from earlier surgery.

Recent evidence indicates most women who opt for no breast reconstruction after a mastectomy report being satisfied with their decision and the results. However, as many as 1 in 4 also reported that their decision to go flat was not supported by their surgeon. If the woman you care about chooses to go flat, you could be a critical source of support for her decision if her medical team seems to be opposed to this decision.

If she forgoes reconstruction, she can request what the National Cancer Institute refers to as *aesthetic flat closure*. It is estimated that as many as 1 in 10 women who choose to go flat wake up from surgery with unsightly, uncomfortable layers of excess tissue, folds, and other small bulges at the mastectomy site. Rather than being smooth and flat, her chest could be left with strange layers and puckered skin, which even someone proud to be flat would consider unsightly. If your wife or partner or friend or relative requests aesthetic flat closure, you can print out "Flat is Beautiful" brochures or images that she can show her surgeon (see, for example, https://notputtingonashirt.org). If the surgeon who will perform the mastectomy seems unsure about achieving acceptable results, encourage her to ask for consultation with a plastic surgeon who is specially trained to create an aesthetically pleasing appearance.

Following going flat surgery, there are other choices she can make. She may adopt a new flat chest appearance, including tattoos across the chest that may please her. When dressed, she may continue to go flat or choose breast forms – prosthetics – worn over the skin but under her clothes to lend the outward appearance of breasts. Most lingerie sections include multiple bra options with pockets for prostheses readily available in stores or online. These can be pinned in place to help ensure they do not shift during normal movements. Women who choose to wear breast forms can select different clothing styles to disguise the lack of cleavage associated with normal breasts, including swimsuits.

Because you care about her, you need to support her choice among the options available to her. Our love for another human being should not be negatively affected by whether she opts for a flat chest, wears a prosthesis under her clothes, or has surgically reconstructed breasts. If she chooses an outward appearance of going flat, be sure you understand her reasons and support her decision. Well-meaning family and friends can sometimes appear unsympathetic by proclaiming their own ideas about femininity, identity, and what *they* believe she should do. You may be called upon to explain to them, in private, how strongly you both feel that this is her decision, deserving of their respect.

Other women do regard reconstructed breasts as important for their well-being. Each year in the U.S., for example, more than 100,000 women undergo breast reconstruction surgery. If her breast-conserving surgery involved removing a proportionately large amount of tissue along with the cancer, she may be offered partial breast reconstruction. Practical considerations about her appearance can also play a role in choosing breast reconstruction, such as concern about prostheses inadvertently slipping out of place and embarrassing her in public. She may want to wear the kind of swimsuits she has always worn, and she may enjoy wearing dresses that show cleavage when dining out and at special social events where this is appropriate. A breast form cannot provide cleavage whereas reconstructed breasts usually do. She could also elect nipple reconstruction surgery and/or nipple tattoos for a more natural appearance. Alternatively, she may purchase custom-made prosthetic nipples with the appearance of natural nipples that can be put on and taken off whenever she wishes. If you are her partner, your support through this decision-making process can have a major impact on her, your relationship, and long-term satisfaction for both of you. She should not be made to feel ashamed about wanting breast reconstruction any more than others who choose to go flat.

If she is inclined towards choosing breast reconstruction, it is important for her to be realistic about likely results. Reconstruction will not create breasts identical to the breasts lost to cancer. They are unlikely to mirror the perfection of Hollywood stereotypes that can create unrealistic expectations. Nor will reconstructed breasts feel the same or be sensitive to touch. Some sensation may return over time, but there is typically a permanent loss of the skin sensitivity and sexual arousal associated with natural breasts and nipples. You and she can view the many before-and-after photographs of breast reconstruction surgeries available online to get a sense of what to expect. Some of these photos will reveal excellent results, more will be average and acceptable, and others will be disappointing. It may be helpful for you to look with her at the results of different breast reconstruction surgeries to prepare both of you for possible outcomes. While she is making this decision, this could also be a good time to take a few photographs of her breasts before surgery, as these photos could be useful in guiding future plastic surgery and/or nipple tattoos.

Types of Reconstruction Surgery

Breast reconstruction most often begins in conjunction with mastectomy surgery while she is still under general anesthesia. Typically, the mastectomy surgeon completes removal of breast tissue, and then the reconstructive plastic surgeon takes over. There may even be two different operating tables set up in the operation theater for the two procedures. One advantage of doing immediate reconstruction is avoiding a second major surgery and concomitant recovery time for the reconstruction. Also, no matter how prepared she felt for the mastectomy, the emotional reaction of waking up from surgery with her breasts missing could be far more negative than she anticipated.

Alternatively, breast reconstruction surgery can be initiated weeks, months, or even years later following recovery from her mastectomy. This option gives her additional time and opportunity to decide whether she wants reconstruction. It may also be the only option available in a hospital or region where the coordination of plastic surgery requires scheduling so far in advance that the mastectomy to treat her cancer would be delayed unacceptably. If she has been a smoker, her oncologist may recommend scheduling reconstruction for a future date after she stops smoking in preparation for that surgery. Smoking tobacco reduces the blood supply to the skin, and even vaping and e-cigarettes have been shown to cause problems with wound healing. Her oncology team may consider these risks unacceptable reasons for delaying life-saving mastectomy surgery to remove cancerous tissue, but prefer she reduce these risks before further reconstruction surgery.

The different ways surgeons create a reconstructed breast after a mastectomy include inserting an artificial expander or implant, a flap of tissue from another place on her body (called autologous reconstruction), or a combination of the two. Following the mastectomy, the plastic surgeon will perform either (a) a one-stage operation to put in the replacement implant immediately; or (b) a two-stage operation that begins with the insertion of an expandable bag containing a small amount of saline solution (sterile salt water) that will be replaced later by an implant filled with silicone or saline designed to last ten years or more. The implant will be positioned either under a chest muscle or over chest wall muscles, and to do this the surgeon will go through the same incision already made for the mastectomy. Either procedure will involve adding a sub-pectoral (under the chest muscles) layer of tissue or mesh reconstruction under the breast to create a kind of sling that will hold the implant in place. Because this may involve the use of human cartilage or other tissue, the plastic surgeon will explain this to her and give her the opportunity to raise any objections or preference for an alternative, artificial mesh material.

Before the reconstruction, the woman will be asked for her preferred breast size following surgery and given options for either cone-shaped or circular shaped implants. There are variations of artificial implants and a dozen different autologous tissue reconstructions, but we present the basics here so you can be better informed. In addition, a helpful and comprehensive website about breast reconstruction surgery in the U.S. can be found at https://www.breastcancer.org/treatment/surgery/reconstruction. Two authoritative sources for information in the UK are: https://www.cancerresearchuk.org and https://www.nhs.uk/conditions/breast-cancer/treatment/#surgery.

Worldwide information on the latest developments in breast reconstruction including up-to-date presentations by international experts is available at https://ecancer.org/en/video?keyword=breast%20reconstruction&template=basic.

Artificial Implant Reconstruction

If her plastic surgeon inserts an implant expander, her chest will initially look flatter and somewhat oddly shaped after the surgery. Beginning with a series of outpatient visits about a month after the mastectomy, the plastic surgeon will "expand" the implant under her skin with scheduled injections of additional saline through a port in the expander. This process is necessary to allow remaining skin to stretch and adapt to gradual increases, as she will have lost skin over her breasts as part of the mastectomy. The plastic surgeon is likely to give her a choice between implants the same size or smaller than her original breast size, but not larger. Once the agreed breast size is reached through the saline injections, outpatient surgery will be scheduled to remove the expander and replace it with a silicone implant. The final surgery usually requires general anesthesia but is considered minor compared with the mastectomy and initial reconstruction surgery. This "swapping over" surgery may be performed in less than an hour, and she will be ready to go home that same day. Pain will be minimal as this is less invasive skin incision surgery, generally healing far more quickly than surgery involving removal of major organs and tissues.

Alternatively, if the more permanent silicone implant was inserted at the time of the original mastectomy surgery, her follow-up visits will entail only check-ups with the mastectomy surgeon and the plastic surgeon to monitor for possible complications during healing.

Autologous or Flap Reconstruction

Autologous tissue flap breast reconstruction procedures are performed less often in comparison with implant reconstruction, for two reasons. Firstly, these require specialized skills not available everywhere. Equally important, flap reconstruction involves removing healthy tissue from elsewhere on her body – hence referred to as autologous – so it's a more invasive surgical reconstruction procedure compared with artificial implants. There will be at least one other major incision on her body, so this may not be a viable choice for women at higher risk of complications due to factors such as age, overall health, or other medical conditions. On the other hand, follow-up research shows more pleasing aesthetics, higher satisfaction, and longer-lasting results from tissue flap reconstructions compared with artificial implants.

In an autologous reconstruction, a "flap" of tissue is taken from another part of her body: this could be her abdomen, buttocks, thighs, back, and flanks (e.g., "love handles," the excess fat on the sides of one's lower waist and back). A flap of donor tissue including blood vessels (perforators), skin, fat, and/or muscle is shifted from another part of her body to her chest then shaped into reconstructed breasts. DIEP, Stacked DIEP, SGAP, Stacked/Hybrid GAP, Latissimus Dorsi, PAP, SIEA, and TRAM flaps all involve transplanting blood vessels, generally along with skin, fat, and sometimes muscle tissue. IGAP, Stacked/hybrid GAP, and Body Lift Perforator flaps require specialized microsurgical expertise that is not available everywhere. Complicated microsurgery to reconnect blood vessels from another part of the body to those in the chest also means longer surgery times, so this may not be viable for women with other health issues. Techniques such as DIEP, Stacked DIEP, SIEA, and TRAM procedures do not involve damage to muscles. Thus, recovery times are quicker with fewer complications, and they do not risk long-term loss of muscle strength at donor sites. Some procedures provide only enough tissue for one breast (e.g., Stacked DIEP, Stacked/Hybrid GAP) whereas others work for reconstructing both breasts (e.g., IGAP, Body Lift Perforator). Certain flap reconstructions will not work for very thin women, larger breasts, and/or women who have had previous surgery such as a C-Section or hysterectomy. Other procedures may be so new there are no long-term data on outcomes, such as Fat Grafting using liposuction to shape fat from the thighs, belly, and buttocks into breasts. More information about tissue flap reconstruction is available at https://www.breastcancer.org/treatment/surgery/reconstruction/types/autologous.

Advantages and Disadvantages of Reconstruction Types

There are advantages and disadvantages to both implant and tissue reconstructions. Both tissue flap and artificial implant reconstructions can be repeated in future surgeries if the original procedure fails in some way. Long-term outcomes favor tissue flaps over artificial implants. If done well and there are no complications, they may never need further attention.

Because they are expected to last a lifetime, tissue flap reconstructions may be preferable for younger women especially. There is some evidence that women and their partners report higher sexual satisfaction over time. The results of tissue flap reconstruction will be more stable and look more natural aesthetically.

The less invasive implant reconstruction is an easier surgery to perform and has shorter operative and recovery times. There is no damage to muscles and other tissue at donor sites elsewhere on her body. Implants can be removed easily if there are complications such as a rupture or an implant failure. Silicone implants generally require surgical replacement after about ten years, involving slightly less recovery time in comparison with the original mastectomy. She can avoid the risk of serious health complications from implant ruptures that could allow silicone to invade surrounding tissues by choosing a saline-filled implant instead; leaking saline is harmless and would simply be absorbed by the body. Implants are more affordable and safer for women who are at increased risk because of age and other health factors.

Tissue flap reconstruction usually means longer surgery times (up to 10 hours under general anesthesia) and longer recovery times for the woman, though some types such as Latissimus Dorsi surgery may take only 3–4 hours. Certain flap reconstructions can mean a permanent loss of muscle strength in the buttocks, back, belly, and thighs. After a TUG procedure, the woman will lose altogether the use of the muscle that pulls the leg upwards towards the body.

There are also other complications associated with tissue flap reconstructions. Some are very recent, so there is less information on long term outcomes. There may not be a plastic surgeon in your region with expertise and experience to perform some of the newest techniques that require complex microsurgery to reconnect tiny blood vessels. In addition, because flap reconstruction "borrows" tissue from elsewhere on her body, she will have at least two incisions to recover from and two wounds to care for. Indeed, TRAM flap surgery results in three incisions – in the chest, lower abdomen, and by her belly button. If she does have flap reconstruction surgery, your help could be essential in caring for a donor incision site on her back or thighs – places on her body she cannot see to monitor closely during the healing process.

Surgery Decisions, Preparation, and Coming Home

Breast reconstruction is major surgery requiring preparation and follow-up, and your assistance can be crucial. Whether reconstruction begins at the same time as her mastectomy or a few months later, preparations for going to the hospital for surgery will be almost identical to those we outlined in Chapter 9 in Box 9.2 "Preparations for Going to the Hospital for Surgery" (pp. 128–129). You can help her with preparations by checking that she receives written instructions from the hospital and reviewing these with her. In addition, Box 9.3 "Coming Home from the Hospital" (pp. 136–139) includes detailed information about things to do before going to the hospital so you and she will be ready when she returns home. These include how to care for her incisions and drains but also making changes at home for her well-being and comfort in the days, weeks, and even months after the surgery.

There may be additional considerations depending upon whether her breast construction surgery involves an implant or a tissue flap from her own body. For example, Luanna and Megumi's plastic surgeons each performed a two-stage implant involving several additional visits after the mastectomy to inject saline into the expander. The first visit was about a month after surgery with two further injections spaced about two weeks apart. Once the agreed breast size was reached, they then had a pre-operation visit several weeks after the third and final saline injection followed by the final implant surgery. As indicated previously, this *swapping over* surgery to remove expanders and replace them with more natural looking and longer-lasting silicone implants is done on an outpatient basis. There will be little pain or discomfort, and recovery after a final implant exchange does not require nearly the same amount of time as the original mastectomy and reconstruction implant surgery.

If her surgery involves a flap reconstruction, there will be the additional caring for the wound and accommodating healing of the tissue flap donor site on her body. She will have more than one wound site to manage and monitor, and if the flap was removed from an area on her body she cannot see easily – such as her back, buttocks, or thighs – you can help by being her eyes to watch for signs of infection. Recovery will take longer for her, so changes in family routines may require months rather than weeks. Results may also include weakened muscles in the donor area that could require permanently changing certain chore responsibilities at home. There will be more frequent visits and consultations with her plastic surgeon to monitor recovery. Depending upon the procedure, the hospital and surgeons will provide detailed instructions about wound care and how to watch for complications. We discuss these later in this chapter.

Costs and Healthcare Coverage

In the U.S., the Women's Health and Cancer Rights Act of 1998 guarantees health insurance coverage for breast reconstruction surgery including nipple reconstruction following mastectomies, whether due to a diagnosis of cancer or to reduce risk associated with identified genetic mutations. Medicare also generally covers breast reconstruction procedures, including nipple reconstruction, but Medicaid coverage varies from state to state. If her insurance policy quibbles about paying for nipple reconstruction surgery, you can help her by finding out as much as you can from the plastic surgeon's office to make the case that this is medically necessary as part of the breast reconstruction. If the health insurance provider considers an operation such as nipple reconstruction to be purely cosmetic, costs may not be covered, and she would have to pay. Wherever you live, you can support her by finding out the costs of the different surgery choices. Even if her insurance or Medicare covers the major portion of a procedure, there is likely to be a required co-pay contribution. In other countries such as Australia and the UK, reconstruction plastic surgeries after a mastectomy are likely to be covered by private insurers and the national health services unless they are judged to be solely cosmetic.

When complications lead to a reoperation such as the removal and replacement of an implant, cost may also come into the decision-making process. An example of surgery that an insurer might consider purely aesthetic would be to minimize a minor symmetry between the woman's two breasts. This is less likely to be covered by insurance, whereas a reoperation to remove an infected tissue expander or diseased flap tissue would be covered. Where the surgery has resulted in an extremely unsightly scar – as can happen with surgery without reconstruction as well – corrective surgery should be covered across the U.S. because the 1998 legislation includes medical interventions related to the woman's mental health and well-being.

Timing and Implications of Adjuvant Treatments

Treatment for cancer generally involves additional therapies in addition to the mastectomy, referred to as *adjuvant therapies* (discussed in more detail in Chapter 9). If her surgery was a bilateral prophylactic mastectomy due to the presence of a genetic mutation highly predictive of cancer, there will be no adjuvant therapies as there was no breast cancer. Thus, breast reconstruction will be offered at the same time as the mastectomy.

When she has cancer and reconstruction is planned, her oncology team is likely to advise additional therapies. Chemotherapy and/or radiation therapy are most likely to be done prior to reconstruction surgery. Recovery after breast reconstruction takes at least four weeks for implants and longer for tissue flaps. Such delays could be considered unacceptable for treating her cancer – particularly if it is later stage and/ or an aggressive type such as triple-negative – whenever her oncology team recommends more than one treatment.

Radiation may be focused on her lymph nodes and not the breasts. If radiation treatment is directed to her breast area, this may happen before reconstruction to avoid negative effects on the reconstructed breast. However, recent treatment developments have demonstrated more acceptable results in terms of feasibility, cosmetic appearance, and sufficiently low complication rates even if radiation is performed at the time of reconstruction. When radiation therapy to the breast area follows a mastectomy, it may be delivered either to the temporary tissue expander or to the replacement silicone implant. Follow-up studies reveal better aesthetic results when radiation is delivered to the expander, but failure rates for the implant are lower when radiation is delayed until after the silicone implant is in place.

If her treatment included adjuvant chemotherapy, radiation can also be prescribed either before or after the expander is swapped for the artificial implant. Radiation may also be part of her treatment plan when she intends to undergo autologous flap reconstruction following the mastectomy, rather than an implant. There is some evidence of increased risk of fat necrosis in women who underwent radiation following flap reconstruction, but this is regarded as inconclusive at the time of this writing. Nevertheless, post-mastectomy radiation of the breast area is problematic for women undergoing breast reconstruction. Thus, radiation is most likely to be prescribed only for women at higher risk of a recurrence or metastatic cancer, such as when cancer is found in her lymph nodes.

Her oncologist and plastic surgeon will be her best source of advice regarding whether and which adjuvant treatments are needed and how they should be sequenced.

Nipple Reconstruction Surgery and Tattoos

If the nipple and areola are removed as part of the mastectomy, there are different options to recreate or simulate them. The simplest is to opt for a nipple tattoo. The permanent 3D nipple tattoos produced by an experienced and specialized nipple tattoo artist are flat to the touch, but the nipple and areola tattoos they create have all the appearance of being three-dimensional. Some women consider the cosmetic results from non-invasive tattoo procedures better than those achieved by nipple reconstruction. The tattoo can include fine details like shading and coloring to resemble what real nipples and areola look like, whereas surgical ones require follow-up tattooing to add color and achieve similar results. The tattoos can even create the illusion of the little bumps on the areola (called Montgomery glands).

Nipple tattooing is a final stage of breast reconstruction and should not be done for at least four months following the final breast or nipple reconstruction surgery. She will want to be sure the nipple is positioned in the right place, and this will not be known until after her breasts have fully recovered from the surgery. A nipple tattoo is not a viable option if radiation treatments have damaged the skin on her breast or the skin is too thin, if she has lymphedema involving her chest, or if she has a history of infections in that area of her body.

She should have the approval of her plastic surgeon for a nipple tattoo. The plastic surgeon can also provide references to licensed tattoo artists who have done good work for others. If she wishes, encourage her to ask to see photos of previous work by the artist she is considering. If she has photos of her own breasts prior to the mastectomy and would like visually similar results, encourage her to show the tattoo artist those photos of how her nipple and areola looked before surgery. Nipple tattoos can be applied at a plastic surgeon's office, in the hospital, or at a nipple tattoo artist's studio. Often the tattoo artist is willing to travel to the plastic surgeon's office or hospital to do the tattooing.

Nipple reconstruction surgery is more complicated than a tattoo. She may prefer its cosmetic results especially if she follows up later by having a tattoo artist add color and an areola to make the nipple look more natural. The main advantage of a nipple reconstruction is that it will project outward from the breast like a real nipple, whereas a tattoo is flat. Nipple reconstruction is usually done on an outpatient basis using skin from the breast area where the nipple will be built, and an areola can be added with a skin graft from another part of the body like the lower belly or from a healed mastectomy or C-section scar. If hers was a partial mastectomy and the nipple on her remaining breast is large enough, the plastic surgeon can remove a portion of that nipple and use it to build the new nipple on her reconstructed breast. The surgeon will take care to match them, and, again, an areola can be added later by a tattoo artist.

Because the reconstructed nipple tends to flatten over time, the plastic surgeon will initially build a larger one. She should talk with the plastic surgeon about how she prefers reconstructed nipples to look; ideally, she will have those photos of how she looked prior to the mastectomy surgery that she can share.

Nipple reconstruction surgery carries a risk of failure and infection, such as a breakdown of tissue because of an inadequate blood supply to the new nipple. If this occurs, a part will need to be cut away (e.g., the tip) or the entire nipple may need to be surgically removed. If the nipple has flattened unacceptably, the plastic surgeon can later use tissue from another part of her body to create more projection once again, secured in place with stitches. An excellent source for up-to-date information on nipple reconstruction and tattooing in the U.S. can be found at https://www.breastcancer.org/treatment/surgery/reconstruction/types/nipple.

Box 10.1 includes more detailed information on how you can help her prepare for and follow up after nipple reconstruction surgery.

Side Effects and Complications

Breast reconstruction may not be a permanent fix, and it is important to monitor for subsequent side effects and complications. Recent data indicate that one in three women who undergo breast reconstruction will experience complications within three years of their mastectomies; one in five will require additional surgery. Yet, reconstruction fails completely in only 5% of cases. Artificial implants are associated with fewer complications compared with autologous tissue flaps. Depending upon the location of the donor site and whether muscles were cut or damaged by the procedure, tissue flaps can result in long-term muscle weakness in the donor area of her body.

Several factors increase the risks of post-operative complications, such as age, not being physically fit, having a pre-existing health condition like diabetes, and tobacco use. Women who undergo a bilateral reconstruction experience more complications than those who underwent reconstruction of one breast only. Having had either chemotherapy or radiation therapy during or after the reconstruction is also associated with more difficulties.

Artificial Implant Side Effects and Complications

Implants may last up to ten years, but they are not permanent. Silicone or saline-filled implants will need to be replaced at some point in the future. This could be sooner rather than later if there are complications such as an implant rupture, implant displacement, or capsular contracture (see below). Implants can become infected, cause infection in surrounding tissue, and be rejected by her body. Symptoms of infection

Box 10.1   Preparation and Follow Up for Nipple Reconstruction and Tattooing

What Happens Before and During

- If you have a photo of her nipples before her mastectomy, show it to the plastic surgeon and/or the tattoo artist. Plastic surgeons often photograph reconstruction work, so if she doesn't have her own photos, she could ask if they have one to use as a guide.
- Encourage her to check with a member of the oncology team to obtain a list of instructions to prepare for the procedure if they have not already given her one. The instructions will differ depending upon whether local or general anesthesia will be used. General anesthesia is not used for tattooing but could be for a nipple reconstruction.
- During an office consultation prior to surgery or tattooing, the plastic surgeon and/or nipple tattoo artist will identify the place on her breasts with markings to show where to make the incisions. It is important for her to be standing when this happens to mark the appropriate location.
- On the day of the surgery or tattooing, help her pick out clothing that she will be comfortable wearing afterwards. This will most likely be a two-piece outfit with a loose-fitting, front-buttoning top. As in previous hospital procedures, make plans for transportation to and from the hospital or clinic and look after any valuable personal belongings during the procedure.
- If her nipple reconstruction is done using local anesthetic, the area where the nipple will be constructed will be numbed by injection. If skin is being taken from another part of her body for a graft, that location will also be numbed. If you know she is likely to be anxious about this, encourage her to ask about a relaxant to help her remain calm.
- If the reconstruction is performed under general anesthesia, an IV line will be inserted and taped in place on her hand or arm, and she will be administered a relaxant through the line prior to surgery.
- She should expect the surgery to take up to an hour.
- Nipple tattooing will also require about 30 minutes per nipple. The procedure is not usually painful given the lessened sensation in her reconstructed breasts, but there are exceptions.

Encourage her to speak up if it hurts and ask the tattooist if she can take something for the pain.

What Happens After

- After the surgery, the surgeon will place a nipple shield, shaped like a tiny hat with a wide flat brim, or a protective dressing over the reconstructed nipple. An antibacterial ointment is likely to be applied and prescribed for use at home.
- If she has had general anesthesia, she will be shifted to a recovery room where you may be able to join her. Once she is awake and her vital signs are normal, she will be discharged, and you can take her home.
- Be sure you and she have written instructions about how to care for the protective dressing and any stitches, which will stay in place for several days to a week. She should not shower until after these are removed.
- Because reconstructed breasts initially lack much sensation, she is unlikely to feel pain in the nipple area after the surgery. The area on her body where the tissue graft was taken from will feel tender or even painful for at least a week. Encourage her to ask the doctor for advice about pain relief.
- Nipple tattoos will be covered by a protective dressing and will require a week to 10 days to heal. She will be advised to avoid chlorinated swimming pools, hot tubs, taking a bath, or any sunbathing for several weeks after the tattooing.

include a high fever, breast pain, redness, and swelling. Her doctor may prescribe antibiotics right away, but this is generally not sufficient to clear the infection. Surgery will be needed to remove infected tissue, continuing the antibiotics until the infection is cleared completely. She may be able to have another surgery to replace the implant several months later, after she has healed.

An implant rupture may be obvious or may show only as a slight swelling above the reconstructed breast. This may sometimes be barely perceptible but indicative of a tear in the implant that is allowing silicone to leak into surrounding tissue. Called a *silent rupture,* this requires removal of the implant. In most cases, the plastic surgeon can proceed immediately with swapping over to a new silicone or saline-filled implant.

There is a low risk the implant will shift and end up in the wrong place on her chest, which can be painful. The implant can settle too low, slipping below the bottom fold of her breast. Implants can also settle too far apart from or too close together in the middle of her chest. These displacements are generally the result of mistakes made during the original implant surgery. In some cases she can simply push the implant back into place with her hands, but additional surgery may be needed to reposition the implant or replace it altogether.

Another side effect associated with implants has been called *dynamic distortion*. When the implant is positioned under a chest muscle, her breast skin may stick to that muscle. The result is that when she flexes her chest muscle, her breast may also pop up and down along with the muscle. While this is annoying and looks a bit odd, it generally causes no pain and – if disguised under clothing – can simply be ignored by most women.

Capsular contracture can result from scar tissue that forms around the silicone implant, which is a natural reaction of the human body to an object that it recognizes as something unnatural. If all goes well, the capsule will be soft or perhaps slightly firm: it will not be noticeable and actually helps keep the implant in place. Sometimes, however, the capsule will become hard and dense, tighten, and then squeeze the implant, causing discomfort and even pain. Any previous radiation therapy – particularly if administered after reconstruction – can increase her risk of developing painful capsular contracture but this could also happen to anyone for unknown reasons. Early signs will be increasing firmness or tightness in the breast as soon as a few months after the surgery or years later. In mild cases of capsular contracture, physical therapy can help, and her medical team should be able to recommend a physical therapist who specializes in working with scar tissue problems. For more severe cases, a plastic surgeon may need to perform a capsulectomy to remove the implant and surrounding capsule, then insert a new implant wrapped in what is called an acellular dermal matrix material to discourage formation of a new capsule. Alternatively, an open capsulotomy may be performed to make small incisions in the capsule around the implant and possibly remove part of the capsule, replacing it with that same acellular dermal matrix material. Again, the implant would be replaced with a new one. If capsular contracture comes back again, this indicates that her body is not accepting the artificial implant. She may have to decide whether to go flat or undergo tissue flap reconstruction. As these alternative procedures involve a major shift in what she originally anticipated, your support for her decision about what to do will be important to her.

There is also the risk of something more serious – but uncommon and highly treatable – called breast implant-associated anaplastic large cell lymphoma (BIA-ALCL), a rare type of blood cancer. This occurs most often in women whose breast implants have textured surfaces. The issue has become serious enough that the use of implants with textured surfaces has recently been discontinued altogether in many hospitals and clinics; most plastic surgeons now use only implants with a smooth surface. Surgery is required to remove the textured implant, and she may also need chemotherapy to ensure the cancer does not spread to her lymph nodes. With early diagnosis and treatment, the prognosis for successful treatment and healing is positive. If you or she notice a change in the appearance or feel of the area surrounding her breast such as a swelling or sudden asymmetry, make sure she contacts her plastic surgeon immediately. Seven years after her original breast reconstruction, Luanna noticed a swelling just above one of her breasts. Ultrasound and MRI diagnostics found trace implant fluid around both implants despite no definite evidence of rupture. Because of the increased risk associated with textured implants, her insurance covered swapping over to smooth surface implants; she also chose saline–filled rather than silicone for the new implants.

In the U.S., the FDA recommends regular screening of silicone-filled implants using an ultrasound or MRI to check for implant rupture, even if she has no symptoms. Screening should begin 5–6 years after the implant surgery, then repeated every 2–3 years. You can work with her plastic surgeon to provide the necessary information, so her health insurance commits to covering the cost of these screenings.

Autologous Tissue Flap Side Effects and Complications

The major risk with autologous tissue flap surgery is a breakdown of tissue called *necrosis* which can result in complete flap failure. Initially, her breast skin may turn dark blue or even black, will feel cold to the touch, and open wounds and scabs may appear. She may have a fever and feel sick. There could also be firm lumps of scar tissue in her reconstructed breast, called fat necrosis. Any of these symptoms should alert you to encourage her to contact her doctor immediately. Skin necrosis that is not healing requires surgery to remove the dead tissue, the entire flap may need to be removed, and she may need a graft of healthy skin from another part of her body. After her chest area is completely healed in a few months, the plastic surgeon may perform another flap reconstruction based upon her situation and condition.

With IGAP flap surgery, there is also a small risk of damage during surgery to the sciatic nerve at the tissue donor site. This would lead to sciatica resulting in an intense, sharp pain along the path of her sciatic nerve from her hips and buttocks then down each leg. While the damage is most likely permanent, the pain can be alleviated by cold or hot packs; stretching exercises; over-the-counter pain medication; and prescription anti-inflammatories or muscle relaxants. Physical therapy is a major source of relief, and you can help by locating a trained professional and following procedures to ensure this is covered by your health insurance. Steroid injections such as cortisone shots can also help temporarily.

The long-term effects can be cosmetically disappointing whenever tissue is sourced from another part of the body. Scars in certain areas on her body may show more than she anticipated. If their appearance bothers her, she may have to change the clothes she wears to hide scars from view. GAP flap surgeries can result in lopsided buttocks when tissue flaps are taken from one side of the body only. You can help by encouraging her to ask about the impact of flap surgeries, not just on the reconstructed breast but also on the part of her body that will be the source for the tissue flap. While the results may still disappoint her, at least when she makes her decision she will be better informed ahead of time about what might happen.

Recovery and Follow-Up

Box 10.2 summarizes advice to support her recovery after breast reconstruction surgery and how to monitor long-term for any complications that may require intervention.

Appearance and Body Image

Research shows that when the woman has a loving, informed, and understanding partner who supports her reconstruction choices, she will feel more positive about her body image and her sexuality. If her partner has conflicted notions about her surgery and has made negative judgments about the results, this will affect not only her but their relationship.

If you as a support person are not actually her husband, her wife (in a same-sex relationship), or her partner but are a friend or family member, you will probably never see the surgical results close-up. But you may know about any worries or concerns she has about her appearance and her future whether she has gone flat or has reconstructed breasts. Your love and reassurance will go a long way towards her adjustment to the new physical reality forced upon her. Now is the time for sincere compliments to be spoken! Tell her she looks nice, tell her the dress or blouse is perfect, and reassure her the swimsuit is "just what the doctor ordered."

Box 10.2   Breast Reconstruction Recovery and Follow-up Advice

Support Before, During, and Right After Reconstruction

- Encourage and help her with lifestyle changes to reduce the risk of complications from surgery and the likelihood of a future implant failure. Pre-existing health conditions cannot be changed, but even a temporary alteration of factors that introduce additional risk can make a difference. You can help her by joining in a plan for losing weight, quitting smoking, and limiting alcohol consumption to reduce risks. Even if she only quits smoking for 4 weeks prior to and for a short time after the surgery, there is evidence this can substantially reduce her risks of reconstruction surgery complications. Sharing this burden will make it easier on her.

- Keep that cancer-calendar we mentioned earlier, on which you and she record all key appointments and commitments. Ensure new appointments and commitments are checked against existing ones.

- Once a week, review the latest written instructions from her medical team regarding upcoming appointments and procedures. Highlight these on the calendar and do your best to rearrange your schedule so you can accompany her, including working with her to organize childcare if needed. If you cannot take time off work for a particular appointment, check with her to see who you can ask to step up to accompany her. There will be friends and family happy to help by covering some of these commitments, so don't hesitate to ask them.

- On the day of an appointment with anyone on her oncology team, discuss with her what issues and questions she has and how you can help support her. Write some key words on a note card to remind you both what she would like to ask the doctor or nurse and have this handy during the appointment. Check it before you leave to remind you both of important issues. But if she chooses to not ask about something on the list during an appointment, remember it is not your role to take charge and ask the questions. Chances are she has a good reason why she did not ask something, so trust her.

- Accompany her to and from hospital visits and other medical appointments, doing the driving when needed. Be sure you yourself are ready to depart on time – do not be the person who must be reminded it is time to leave for the hospital! Check first thing in the morning that both your cellphones are fully charged and, if they are not, get this done. She has enough on her mind!

- When you get return home after each visit, pamper her a little. She is likely to want to take a sponge bath or shower if permitted following appointments and procedures, so create space and free time for her to do this. After she has had time to relax, bring out your list of queries and discuss updates – you don't have to hit her with this the minute you both arrive home! Plan a special meal that evening which you (and possibly even the children) will prepare, or you could organize her favorite take-home meal.
- After her final surgery is over, celebrate! She is still recovering physically, so this will most likely be a quiet event or loving time together rather than a wild and crazy party. She may feel like calling her mom, dad, a grown-up child, or a good friend to talk on the phone. You can discuss something special you can do once she is feeling well again. Resist the temptation to decide what this should be and instead bend to her preferences – there will be plenty of other times when you will get your way! Then, after you know what she wants, follow up and plan to make it happen several months later – put it on that calendar.

Support During Year Two to Year Ten After Reconstruction

- Keep up the calendar you started last year, and make sure it includes the first-year follow-up appointment dates and times with her oncologist and plastic surgeon (perhaps two appointments with each doctor, six months apart). Plan to go with her to these biannual appointments or check if she would appreciate having a friend or other family member be the one to come along. You will both be keeping a watchful eye for any complications, but on the day before each appointment, go over anything she would like to ask and make one of those short lists again for the doctor and nurse.
- During years 3–5 following surgery, her appointments will likely spread out more and may be scheduled once every 8 months or even once a year. After five years, her appointments are likely to be only once a year. After several more years

with no complications, she will probably be told she can have regular doctor visits if she wishes but otherwise to just call with any concerns. Keep up your awareness of possible side effects or complications, including any signs of a recurrence of cancer, ongoing pain, muscle weakness, tissue disease, and signs of infection or other complications.

- Because she will be going less frequently for medical check-ups, your support can be crucial in helping to monitor for complications. If she has a silicone implant, watch for subtle changes at or near the breast reconstruction that could reveal a leakage of silicone material from a rupture or tear in the implant which could compromise her immune system. If you notice something different about the shape of her chest near her breast, encourage her to make an appointment with her oncologist and plastic surgeon immediately. Encourage her to request an ultrasound or MRI to check for possible silent impact rupture.

You may be the one to volunteer to go shopping with her to find some attractive new clothes that fit the new her. It may have been many months since she was able to or had any enthusiasm for trying on clothes, so break the ice. Encourage her to take the first steps and pick out something to wear for an upcoming special event or just for walks around the block. She may want you to go shopping with her or she may prefer to reach out to another woman close to her who could help. It will be important to be sure your loved one agrees to you approaching them. She will know whom to approach – she may love them all dearly, but not everyone she knows will necessarily be her first-choice shopping companion! Remember, others may be reluctant to offer and not quite sure what to do, so, if she agrees, let them know how much they will be appreciated for help like this.

Sexual Relationships and Sexuality

One area that has been relatively under-researched until recently is the sexual satisfaction of a woman and her intimate partner after a mastectomy and breast reconstruction. Over time, there will be more restoration of feeling and skin sensitivity following breast reconstruction. But this is most likely to be minimal in comparison to a woman's natural sexual response from stimulation of her nipples and breasts. Consequently, some couples report difficulties achieving sexual arousal, and women report lessened breast sensation, vaginal lubrication, and ability to achieving orgasm following a mastectomy with breast reconstruction. The evidence to date indicates that immediate reconstruction leads to better sexual outcomes than delayed reconstruction, and that autologous breast reconstruction results in greater satisfaction sexually than artificial implants. Nipple sparing and reconstruction surgery can also enhance sexual satisfaction, though the positive physical effects are reported to be small. Reoperations also put the woman at risk for more negative sexual outcomes.

There are exciting new developments in plastic surgery that could alter unfavorable sexual sensitivity outcomes for many women and their partners. *Neurotization* is a new technique being trialed in TRAM, DIEP, and SIEA tissue flap surgery. It involves connecting a cutaneous nerve from the abdominal tissue flap to the anterior branch of the third intercostal nerve between the woman's sternum and her third rib. This innovative surgery is not available everywhere but may be available in your region, and she may be eligible for this approach. Our sources are from 2020 and 2021 research reports published by expert medical teams in the U.S. and the UK (the references are listed at the end of this chapter). By the time you read this, there is likely to be more information about these kinds of plastic surgeries. You can investigate by doing a search online using the term *neurotization* to update for more current developments.

This research is important for sexual outcomes but also for other reasons directly related to her physical health. Reconstructed breasts that are less sensitive to touch – and may even seem numb – will be more susceptible to thermal and other kinds of injuries. Her skin over the reconstructed breasts will be at risk for sunburn, for example, even under her swimsuit. On your next visit to the grocery store or pharmacy, locate a good quality sunscreen for sensitive skin (something marked for use on the face is good) with a high SPF rating for her to apply on her breasts when sunbathing and/or swimming.

Sexual outcomes can be affected by factors other than the type and timing of the surgery. Older women report more positive sexual outcomes than younger women, but this may be attributable to factors other than age such as how long they have been with their partner, how confident they are in the relationship, how comfortable they are in communicating with their partner (having had longer to develop stronger strategies), placing less importance on physical appearance ideals in comparison with those who are younger, and even having developed – over time – more varied sexual repertoires to access with their partners for sexual arousal and to achieve orgasm.

If you are her intimate partner, what has also been shown to be most important is your relationship and how you and your intimate partner interact. If you had relationship and marital problems prior to her surgery, these difficulties do not go away after a mastectomy followed by her either going flat or undergoing breast reconstruction. You may benefit from couples counseling, preferably with a professional who has experience both with cancer and with providing sexuality advice – or can make a referral for you. Your healthcare provider may be able to suggest a few possibilities.

The best news of all is there are other things you and she can do throughout this experience that are related to improved outcomes. If you are supportive and knowledgeable about what she is going through, that helps. As her partner, your involvement in helping to make and then supporting her treatment decisions is crucial. You and she are not to blame if sexual relations are less satisfying and harder work than they were before the cancer. But the good news is that you and she will experience better postoperative sexual outcomes by continuing to work together to support one another.

Summary and Recommendations

- Not every woman chooses breast reconstruction after a mastectomy, so be open to understanding how she feels about whether to go flat or to undergo breast reconstruction.
- Before she meets with her oncologist to review her decisions about surgery, offer to find out additional, up-to-date information about options such as aesthetic flat closure, immediate or delayed reconstruction, and the different types of implants. We list relevant websites at the end of this chapter help you begin your search.
- Know that couples' satisfaction with mastectomy and breast reconstruction outcomes is greatly influenced by your own knowledge about the procedures, your understanding of how she feels about what is happening to her, and your ability to communicate openly with her. Especially if you are her wife in a same-sex relationship or her husband, be consistent in offering to share in the decision-making while always leaving the final choices up to her.
- Make certain you and she understand the sequencing and timing of additional treatments such as chemotherapy and radiation in relationship to breast reconstruction surgery. Encourage her to ask her plastic surgeon and oncologist to explain anything that is unclear.
- Keep two copies of any written instructions given to her by her oncology team and at the hospital or clinic where procedures take

place – one for you and one for her. Encourage her to read these through right away when they are given to her, asking the care nurse for clarification if she or you have any questions. Read them through again after you both return home, as well as before and after any procedure related to her operation, wound care, bandaging, and treatment side effects to monitor. Whenever you can, watch the nurse dressing her wound, so you know how to do this.

- Review again Boxes 9.2 Preparations for Going to the Hospital for Surgery and Box 9.3 Coming Home from the Hospital in Chapter 9 prior to her breast reconstruction operation, whether it is immediate and begun during the mastectomy or delayed and performed months later. She will appreciate the things you can do to support her, but always ask what she would like before you jump in!

- Although most costs associated with breast reconstruction are covered by health insurance, Medicare, and Medicaid in the U.S., national health care services in the UK and elsewhere, and private insurers in many countries, not all procedures may be covered. With her consent, you can help by checking what will be covered and working with her plastic surgeon to justify procedures in advance of surgery to increase the chances of coverage. You can find out the costs of any co-pays that will be required, so these can be anticipated, and you can help plan for them in advance.

- Try not to have unrealistic expectations about how her reconstructed breasts will look after the surgery, how they will feel, and – if you are her partner – how satisfied you and she will be with the results. There may be disappointments but appreciate how breast reconstruction can enhance her well-being and sense of her feminine self. Do not be stingy with compliments when she looks beautiful!

- If she is offered different options for artificial implants versus tissue flap surgery, review the advantages and disadvantages with her and encourage her to seek clarification from the plastic surgeon with questions and concerns prior to making her final decision.

- Clarify your own feelings about nipple-sparing surgery and tattoos even as you pledge to support her decision about these options.

- Help her monitor for side effects and complications, not just during the timeframe of her surgery but long into the future. If she has a silicone implant, she will need to be on the watch for complications that may not occur for years but can have serious implications for her health. Make a reminder for you both somewhere you won't miss. If your healthcare provider does not call her in for a check on her implant after 5-6 years, encourage her to take the initiative and schedule an appointment.

- Anticipate that a silicone implant will need to be removed and replaced at least once in future years, and that this is normal. At the time, encourage her to check that the replacement implant is not textured and that she has a choice between silicone and saline-filled.
- Be open to seeking help and support from others in the family and your friendship networks. Another family member or friend may be in the best position to help her with shopping or just to talk about her experiences: try not to think you must do everything. She will value your caring and concern, but it will also make her happy to know that you both have support from others who love her as well.

Sources for More Information

https://www.medicare.gov/coverage/breast-prostheses (discusses Medicare Part B, Medical Insurance)

https://www.youtube.com/watch?v=sqYzPbGBCOI (an overview of mastectomy/breast reconstruction by Johns Hopkins Hospital professionals)

Al-Ghazal, S. K., Fallowfield, L., & Blamey, R. W. (2000). Comparison of psychological aspects and patient satisfaction following breast conserving surgery, simple mastectomy and breast reconstruction. European Journal of Cancer, 36, 1938–1943.

Baker, J. L., Dizon, D. S., Wenziger, C. M., Streja, E., Thompson, C. K., Lee, M. K., DiNome, M. L., & Attai, D. J. (2021). ASO Visual Abstract: "Going Flat" after mastectomy: Patient-reported outcomes by online survey. Annals of Surgical Oncology, 28, 2507. 10.1245/s10434-021-09769-3

Mak, J. C. K., & Kwong, A. (2019). Complications in post-mastectomy immediate breast reconstruction: A ten-year analysis of outcomes. Clinical Breast Cancer, 20:5, 402–407. 10.1016/j.clbc.2019.12.002

Van de Grift, T. C., Mureau, M. A. M., Negenborn, V. N., Dikmans, R. E. G., Bouman, M.-B., & Mullender, M. (2020). Predictors of women's sexual outcomes after implant-based breast reconstruction. Psycho-Oncology, 29, 1272–1279. 10.1002/pon.5415

Vartanian, E. D., Lo, A. Y., Hershenhouse, K. S., Jacob, L., & Patel, K. M. (2021). The role of neurotization in autologous breast reconstruction: Can reconstruction restore breast sensation? Journal of Surgical Oncology, 123, 1215–1231. 10.1002/jso.26422

11 Telling Family and Friends: Disclosure and Privacy

This chapter focuses on decisions about disclosure and privacy likely to be made by a couple within a family unit, so will be most relevant to you if you are the patient's husband/wife or partner. The information is also relevant, but perhaps less so, to other supporters outside the immediate family. We address the challenges of sharing information about the diagnosis and treatment of breast cancer with others, including suggestions about how, what, and when to tell young children still living at home.

Agreeing About Privacy and Sharing Information

Over time, most couples will have established informally their mutual understanding about how much and what kind of information they share with others. They discuss matters such as when to tell friends and family about upcoming travel; whether to share financial challenges; decisions about buying a new house or moving to another state; changing jobs; and perhaps even private things such as sharing details with a best friend or parent about a marital problem. Most couples with children have probably discussed parenting issues with their own parents, siblings, or other couples who have children at similar ages. If one or both of you is on social media – posting on Instagram, Facebook, and/or Twitter, for example – you generally know when your spouse would be offended by a posting of life events or even photos. Some families have clear guidelines such as agreeing never to post pictures of their young children publicly, outside family and close friends. For others, this is not an issue.

You may even have discussed the boundaries of sharing information about medical conditions. Both men and women are likely to unload their worries, trials, and tribulations about gender-specific conditions with a close friend or sibling of the same sex (e.g., an enlarged prostate in men, hot flashes in women). Ordinarily, your spouse does not mind you

DOI: 10.4324/9781003194088-11

sharing this information with a confidant, someone you trust who is not motivated to repeat private details to others.

Yet, a breast cancer diagnosis – like the diagnosis of any illness with major health and life-threatening implications – is different from the information your family typically shares every day. It is not your place to take charge of telling others about the cancer. If you and your partner disagree about sharing this information, it is the woman with breast cancer who should have the first and last say about whom to tell what level of information and detail. The person with a greater connection to the information must have the greatest influence in how that information is handled and shared. Her views on privacy and disclosure of medical matters could differ from yours. If you as her husband, wife, or support person have never previously discussed this explicitly, now is the time to do so.

We know that women with breast cancer can have extremely divergent views about privacy and disclosure. There are also cultural differences and expectations to consider. Some women are fine with their extended circle of family, friends, co-workers, and even acquaintances knowing they have breast cancer. Some want others to know right away and are comfortable with the offers of support, caring, and sympathy. Your partner may be completely comfortable telling her story to others. On the other hand, both of you may prefer to keep some things private, and you do not want to share personal details that might embarrass her in the future.

She may choose to seek a social support network of other women with breast cancer; after all, this diagnosis may be her only experience and she may not know anyone personally who has had breast cancer. As supportive as you try to be, she may still want to talk with other women who are going through a similar experience. Her medical team and/or hospital clinic may offer information about a local support group for women with breast cancer. She can also ask her nurse if there is another patient in similar circumstances who would be willing to talk with her. Cindy Boss notes how she was asked by a nurse to call another patient who wanted reassurance about an upcoming surgery that she herself had just gone through (see Sources for More Information at the end of this chapter). If your partner seeks other women to talk to, resist the temptation to feel excluded, hurt, or rejected in any way – this is nothing personal!

There will be other choices as well: participation in an online support group has the advantage of being more anonymous and convenient. She can select the place and times that work for her. Online support groups are becoming increasingly popular, and they can help a breast cancer patient cope with her emotions and stressors. By seeking this social support apart from you and her home, she can also shed feelings of sadness, guilt, or stress associated with worry about being a burden to her family – and to you. The social distance of an online support group even gives her an opportunity to complain, anonymously, about something that has upset her without risk of offending you or others in her family!

For other women, however, participation in a support group of breast cancer patients interferes with effective coping. Whether face-to-face or online, group sessions can be aversive if they arouse greater anxiety about the illness and its treatment. Listening to other women tell their stories may be the opposite of calming or comforting! If you notice that she seems more upset or discouraged after attending a group support session or after being online with other breast cancer patients, ask her gently if she wants to talk about these experiences with you. She might want to consider finding a different support group to try.

Some women will prefer to keep their breast cancer experience as private as possible, for different reasons. Sometimes an extreme approach to privacy is driven by feelings of shame or embarrassment about having cancer. This can be a symptom of a larger issue that needs to be addressed: her breast cancer is not her fault, and no woman should be made to feel this way. You may discover that your partner has had a particularly unpleasant experience earlier in her life when she felt demeaned or blamed by a medical professional after seeking advice for a gynecological problem. No woman finds gynecological examinations pleasant – no matter how necessary and important they are – and most women are likely to have strong feelings built up over many years. If you are a man, you will not know what those experiences are like and how they make a woman feel even if the medical team is being their most sensitive. If she shares something with you that has made her feel demeaned or bullied – even if her reaction sounds extreme to you – listen to what she is saying and be sympathetic. You can never "walk in her shoes" where breast cancer is concerned. But you can be a rock in her life, someone she can trust to listen, care, and believe her when she says something is wrong or makes her feel bad.

If you and/or she are religious – or if other family members are religious, even though you are not someone may believe the cancer is God's retribution for past injustices or even punishment for her sins. If anyone in the family blames her for having cancer, you as a support person have a big job to do. You will need to help remedy this situation – both for her and for the insensitive persons responsible for making her feel this way. If she agrees, you could be the one to speak with someone in the family who appears to be blaming her for the cancer. Women with breast cancer should not ever be made to feel they did something to deserve this.

The woman you care about may value being more private about her cancer because of strong biases about identity. She may not want to discuss her diagnosis and treatment with an extended circle. To some women, this would be like allowing cancer to become her identity, to take over who she is in the eyes of others. Nevertheless, she is likely to acknowledge her family has a right to know about the diagnosis and will value their support during difficult times. It is only fair to tell them about circumstances that would inevitably affect their lives as well as hers, both now and possibly even into the future. Yet, she may be less interested in sharing this information with many others outside her immediate family. If you and she usually socialize often with certain friends, they are bound to notice changes in your routines and her appearance. Cutting back on spending time with them without explanation could be driving away good friends exactly when you most need them. As her support person, you will be challenged to respect however she chooses to let others know about her diagnosis and treatment. You can even be especially helpful by rehearsing with her how you should respond to others when they ask questions.

Remember that she should always be given the choice of being the one to tell certain people, sometimes by herself and sometimes together with you. You should both tell your young children together, but who should tell others is something you can let her decide. There will be times when she will be pleased to have you be the one to share information. You should offer to do so whenever she is comfortable with having you do this. But let her do the talking when she clearly prefers to do so and allow her to take the lead even when you tell others together, as a couple.

At the end of the day, she owns the story. You will be an engaged, involved, loving co-author – but it is her story.

Preparation for Sharing Information

It may be helpful for you and your wife or partner to make a list of everyone in your social network – family and friends – who is likely to care and/or feel they have a right to know about her breast cancer. Don't leave anyone out. Go through the list together and agree on whom you will tell and how much to tell. Will you tell friends and, if so, which ones? Will you tell your employers? Will you and she tell your employees if you run a business or have others working for you? Will you tell your child's school?

Whenever possible, information sharing should be face-to-face. You can help by drafting a few sentences for sharing, either by email or written in a card, to provide the essential information she has agreed to tell others. The words can be edited and adapted for different persons by either of you as part of normal communications when the occasion arises. But the basic template would be there, and you will have spared her – and you – the task of repeating oneself, over and over again.

Telling Others

Telling Children and Family

In addition to young children living at home, other close family members will also need to know. Parents and siblings will expect to be told. Telling her parents can be complicated, particularly as her mother and father could react differently. Carson and Cindy Boss recommend telling them as early as possible, not putting it off. She will know how best to do this and if one parent should be told first. Parents usually will want to do everything they can to help, and they may ask for the same information about her medical condition more than once – their emotions are likely to be as intense as your own.

Adult children – who may have families of their own – are another special group of people who need to know what's going on. A son or daughter can also be tremendous help when you need support and someone to be with her when you cannot. If you need a few days off – someone to stay with her when you must travel out-of-town for work or to see family – they can be the perfect person to fill in. They will genuinely appreciate being given the opportunity.

Other relatives further down the list include cousins, aunts, uncles, and so on. If the cancer is hereditary due to genetic causes such as BRCA1 or BRCA2 gene mutations (see Chapter 2, p. 24), she will be advised to tell blood relatives. They may be unaware they could also be carrying those cancer-causing anomalies (see also Chapter 5). Both men and women relatives can be affected and/or pass on the genetic mutations to their own children. These family members will benefit if she not only tells but also gives them a copy of her own genetic counseling report. This will enable them to seek genetic testing and justify insurance coverage testing and counseling costs. Some family members may resist genetics testing because of concerns about privacy and past discrimination that has selectively disadvantaged certain cultural and ethnic groups. If this is an issue, you could help by seeking advice from your health provider about how to handle this.

If yours is a blended family with stepchildren, you must inform your children's other parents and let them know you want to be the ones to tell your children. You may both want to meet together with each of the other parents, so you can support her and help to answer any of their questions and reach understandings about what the children should know.

Schools and Teachers

You should discuss whether to tell your child's school and teachers. If one of your children begins to act out in some way that could be the result of stress or anxiety (see Chapter 12), it could be helpful for you and your wife to speak confidentially to your child's teacher and to a counselor at school. You will want to get the school on board, so they understand what is going on and are alerted to contact you right away when a problem emerges.

Telling Employers, Co-Workers, and Employees

If she works, she will need to tell her employer and selected co-workers. If she runs a business and/or has other employees who report to her at work, employees may also need to be told. Generally, she can delay revealing the cancer and the treatment until schedules conflict, and she may prefer to delay rather than risk negative effects on her career – however inadvertently – if others pass her by, assuming she cannot handle the job or increased responsibility. Similarly, you will have to tell your own employer, some of your co-workers, and your own employees whenever duties at home mean schedule changes and missing time at work.

Eventually, however, both of you will have to share knowledge of the illness and treatment with your employers and others at work. People will be able to help if they know what you and she need and why. Research has found that employers are likely to be sympathetic to the need for occasional changes in schedule given a diagnosis of cancer. Most husbands and partners report their employers accommodate flexible working hours so you can accompany her to medical appointments or chauffeur your children when she cannot do so. Your employer may be generous and even give you permission to leave anytime with minimal notice or at the last minute when you get a call asking for help. Employers are usually sympathetic to changes such as re-directing reporting lines temporarily or setting up different communication mechanisms for times when you or she are unavailable. Finally, if more time off work is needed, the Family and Medical Leave Act in the U.S. entitles both patients and family caregivers access to extended periods of unpaid, job-protected leave for an illness; see https://www.dol.gov/agencies/whd/fmla.

Telling people at work is another communication that should be mutually agreed and timed. You will not want to tell your employer/employees unless and until she has also told her employer/employees – word gets around!

Telling Young Children

One of the most important tasks facing parents when the mother is diagnosed with cancer is the responsibility to tell her (and your) children. There will be many things they want and need to know about what is happening and will happen that can affect them and their lives – not just their mom. The previous section discussed privacy issues that should place the desires of the person with cancer first in decisions made by the family and about information shared with the family. Yet, no matter how private someone prefers to be about cancer, the time will come when there is no way you can avoid telling young children living at home. They are bound to see changes and even pick up on your mood. (See also Chapter 12)

You will have your own worries about what the cancer diagnosis means for her, for you, for your children, and for your lives – all the while hoping everything will be like it used to be once she recovers (see also Chapter 14). You will have occasional if not nagging feelings of inadequacy about whether you are doing the right things to support your partner emotionally and physically. It will be difficult for you to avoid feeling excluded if she is extremely private and does not want to talk about what she's going through. You are likely to worry just as much as she does about whether the cancer will be cured or will come back, and those worries will be exacerbated whenever the news from doctors involves diagnoses of aggressive cancers and cancer in later stages. You may also worry about the financial difficulties such as partial loss of income and the cost of co-pays despite having good health insurance. If you do not have health insurance to cover the lion's share of treatment costs, these financial worries will be major and can involve making hard choices about how to raise funds to pay for treatment.

As important as these issues are to you and no matter how much they dominate your thoughts from week to week, these are not things you want your children to think and worry about (Chapter 12 talks more about this). You and your wife will be working through these issues by yourselves, and you should do your best to make safe spaces for any difficult conversations the two of you need to have privately – apart from the children. Even as you deal with these other issues, a very difficult and important task facing you and her will be deciding what to tell your children, not just what to tell but when to tell, how to tell, and who does the telling. And remember, it's crucial for you both to realize that you cannot protect your children from the cancer diagnosis just as you cannot completely protect yourself from its consequences. It will affect the whole family, and how you react to the cancer and treatment will influence how your family and your children cope and keep strong.

It is OK to wait a few weeks after the diagnosis, but not for long. So now let's imagine it has been a month into chemo, and you both know you cannot keep this secret any longer. She may have cut her hair short in preparation for the inevitable hair loss, she may be looking tired, there could be days when she is unavailable to run errands, and so on. Now is the time they need to know.

When to Tell and What to Say

Children know when something is wrong. They may even sense your anxiety during those days or weeks while you both wait for the results of diagnostic testing – particularly as the testing was done precisely because cancer is suspected. You and she can delay telling very young children (i.e., under age 8) at first, before any prescribed chemotherapy, surgery, radiation, or hospitalizations associated with those treatment options affect the family schedule and make it obvious that mom is ill. We think this is perfectly okay, but it is crucial for both parents to agree when you will share this information. There should be no surprises. Remember also that you are her support person, so she should have more say in these decisions than you. Do not wait so long to tell the children that your telling timetable is lagging behind their fears and worries. After all, you would not want them to hear it from someone other than their mom and dad, and you do not want them to worry but be afraid to ask.

A key message with your children is to communicate openness. Encourage children to ask any questions that are on *their* minds, at any time, then answer the question directly and honestly. There is no need to elaborate further unless they have another question: keep your answers simple and straightforward.

Another key message is that you – the parents – will be the trusted source of information about mom's cancer. This means that you want your children to turn to you whenever anyone else tells them something about breast cancer and/or about their mom's illness. You want to be able to correct misinformation and probably follow-up with someone who you feel has crossed a line in talking with one of your children.

Discussing Changes to Routines

Most moms and dads work outside the home these days, so one of the first things children will notice is a change in work schedules adjusted to accommodate doctor's appointments and treatments like chemotherapy or radiation. Some dads may not be in the habit of doing certain things around the house or chauffeuring for children and other family members. Your kids will notice if you suddenly start doing these things – especially if you have changed your work schedule. Chapter 12 discusses the many changes to family routines that might be needed and how to accommodate them, but here we focus on just a few key issues relevant to that first conversation about the cancer with your children.

Hair loss from chemo will not occur for the first few weeks and your partner may not experience nausea. There could be no visible signs right away that something is wrong. Nevertheless, we advocate telling early is better than later, and there is value in having your children see you preparing for the difficult days ahead, calmly and with resolve to do the best you can. You can begin right from the start to practice constructing *Restorative Narratives* that promote good health and adjustment to life's challenges (see Box 11.1).

Box 11.1   Restorative Narratives for Health Promotion

Stories can provide a useful, informal way to communicate important information about health, illness, hardships, and other challenges in life – all unavoidable parts of life. There is good empirical evidence that stories highlighting hope and resilience are more helpful in promoting positive behavior and attitudes than stories emphasizing suffering or negative emotions. A *Restorative Narrative* is one that focuses on hope and the progression towards recovery during an experience, and information about a mom's breast cancer should be focused on her strengths and how the strengths and contributions of everyone in the family will support her. Restorative Narratives promote resilience which can serve your children well as they go through their lives confronted with future challenges.

(Fitzgerald, Paravati, Green, Moore, & Qian, 2020)

Not too long after the diagnosis, you and she should talk privately about what and how to tell the children. By waiting until after doctors have told you more details and what to expect, you'll be able to share accurate and relevant information with your children about their mom's breast cancer. Pick a time for that first talk when there is no competing commitment for anyone in the family for at least a couple of hours. The middle of a Saturday morning could work well, depending on your typical weekend activities. In contrast, bedtime is probably not an ideal time as children can imagine their worst fears alone in bed right before falling asleep. Pick a location where everyone is reasonably comfortable, sitting around facing one another.

We have listed here some key messages and a sequence to guide your planned Restorative Narrative to tell your children about mom's breast cancer. This is not meant to be a script that you must follow word-for-word. What you say and how you say it to your own children will reflect your approach and how you and she wish to share information with them about the cancer, her treatment, and likely effects on the family.

- Set up the conversation first. Say you will be telling them something important that is going to affect the family now and in the future. Make sure you say this is only the first family conference, and you plan to talk more about this later. You want them to ask questions and talk to either of you as parents any time, with any concerns they may have.
- Before too much suspense and fear builds up, get right to it: "Your mom has breast cancer. The doctors say that...." [here you decide how much to tell but reassure them it is treatable. If this is an early stage, say so. If her cancer is in a later stage where the prognosis is unclear, don't share this yet but emphasize treatment instead].
- Ask your children to tell you what they know about cancer – and about breast cancer specifically. Before you give them new information about their mom's cancer is the time to find out what is already in their heads – what they know and what they think about it. Correct blatant misinformation such as beliefs that everyone dies when they get cancer but avoid details now. Instead, move on to the next point on your list for this family conference.
- Tell them you will tell them the truth, and they should come to you whenever they hear something or whenever anyone else says something to them about this. Tell them lots of people have heard things about cancer, most people have no personal experience, and

only their mom and you know about her cancer. That is why it is important they come to you with questions or concerns.

- Tell the children you are keeping this in the family for now if this is what you and she have agreed. Tell them you are telling only your parents – their grandparents – and other close family members you have decided to tell (e.g., in a blended family, the other parents). If true, say you are telling only very close friends just now, and you hope they will let you know if they want to tell any of their close friends. Mention that mom would like to be a little bit private and not have everyone look at her like she is sick or some kind of victim whenever she does anything or goes anywhere. She wants to be as normal as possible, and cancer is not who she is!
- Talk about family routines. Mention who will be driving them to activities or school whenever schedules are likely to be turned upside down and talk about how they can help (see Chapter 12). You might set up a "tasks" calendar including household jobs that must be done, and they could help decide who will do these for now. A key message here is you both want the family to continue to be as normal as possible. This will include doing special trips and activities together over the coming weeks and months even if they are not as far away and are shorter than originally planned. It will depend on how strong mom is feeling at the time.
- Talk about any temporary changes that will be needed. If surgery is coming up, ask them to think about how the family could temporarily re-arrange bedrooms for just a couple of weeks, so mom can have her own place to recover with uninterrupted sleep. Emphasize this will only be for a couple of weeks – not permanent.
- Tell them you know this is scary news, but mom is strong, she has good doctors, and you both expect she will make a full recovery. Tell them you will worry and may even look sad once in a while, but that too is normal and shows how much you care. On the other hand, you are determined not to let cancer take over the family and define your love for one another. They too may worry sometimes and even be sad, and that's okay. But the family will hang together in being strong for one another – not drag one another down. The message is that Mom needs us to be strong. We have every reason to expect a full recovery and getting through this will make us all stronger in the future.
- Finish by saying something like, "We love you so much. Now let's go do [pick a joint activity, it could even just be lunch] together just like usual!" Over the next few hours, days, weeks, and months, always be honest about the diagnosis, express confidence in the

prescribed treatment choices, emphasize that mom is strong and ready to make the right decisions to be healthy, that you are right beside her and will support her all through this. Stress how important it is that the family tries to be as normal as possible. You will not ignore her cancer, but neither will you make it the center of everything the family does.

Getting Information for Your Children

There is good research evidence that children who are well informed will show better adjustment to a parental cancer diagnosis. There are many available resources about positive strategies for sharing cancer information with older children and with children whose parent has advanced cancer. While less is known about the needs of parents with younger children when the cancer treatment is expected to be curative, there are accessible and child-friendly books you can get for them. Sinclair and her colleagues (2019) in Australia found it helpful to have easily accessible and practical resources for mothers to share, and quantity was not nearly as important to mothers as quality.

Finding children's books and even websites for different age ranges could be a good job for you as the support parent. We recommend you locate good resources for children and have them handy before or shortly after that first talk. This will show them from the beginning that you will be the best source of information about their mom's breast cancer. We have listed several resources at the end of this chapter, but there will be other good books plus new books available in the future. You can search sites such as Amazon and Barnes & Noble Online using key phrases such as "Children's Books about Cancer" and then narrowing down your search to a focus on moms with breast cancer. (There is a URL address in Chapter 12 for the best books for children that could be a good place to start.)

Don't force these books on your children. Instead, wait until you have one or two for each of the age ranges of your children, then as casually as you can take them out and share those you like best. We recommend doing this individually with each child. That way, you can look at the books together without brothers and/or sisters standing around "waiting" while listening passively to what may be an age-inappropriate discussion for them.

With young children who still enjoy having a parent read to them, you could volunteer to read the book either right away or later at the usual time. However, if you do read a "cancer story" book to a child in the evening, be sure to follow up by reading another favorite, short picture book afterwards and before the goodnight kiss. You want to avoid having worries about mom's cancer taking over your child's final thoughts before falling asleep.

Summary and Recommendations

- Open communication between the woman with breast cancer and you as her support person is a crucial aspect of psychological adjustment, emotional well-being, and resilience in facing challenges ahead.

- Address any unresolved issues between you as a couple about who owns the information about her cancer, establishing agreed principles in advance regarding the extent of disclosure versus privacy for her diagnosis and treatment.

- Make a list of who may need to be told and take responsibility to draft a template information-sharing letter or email for both of you to adapt for future use in sharing information with others. Agree that the woman with breast cancer should be given the first option to tell others, but you will take this on if she prefers.

- Support the choice she makes about whether to participate in a breast cancer support group either face-to-face or online, giving her space to communicate without your involvement in additional supports of her choosing.

- Prepare in advance for an initial family conference, together as parents, to tell young children living at home what is happening with their mother, with regular follow-up conversations both with the children individually and as a family.

- Practice and script your Restorative Narratives for talking about the cancer, the treatment, and how you will support and empower the patient and her loved ones to be resilient, no matter what.

- Emphasize to everyone in the family that mom is determined to get better, is receiving excellent treatment, and your resilience will help her to recover with time. In the meantime, despite necessary but temporary changes to routines and responsibilities, it is important for mom and everyone else in the family to feel and behave as normally as possible.

- Ensure your children view you and their mother – their parents – as the authoritative source of information about her cancer and its treatment. Encourage them to tell you and seek your advice whenever someone outside the home speaks with them and may make insensitive and possibly disturbing comments. Follow up by talking privately with anyone close to your family who does this.

- Revisit your information sharing plans and scripts over time to make needed and agreed changes and updates.

Sources for More Information

https://www.cancer.net/coping-with-cancer/talking-with-family-and-friends/how-cancer-affects-family-life (discusses the effects of cancer on partners, friends, and family)

https://www.cancernetwork.com/search?searchTerm=caregivers (discusses the impact of cancer on others)

https://breastcancernow.org/information-support/facing-breast-cancer/telling-family-friends-about-your-breast-cancer (discusses what and how to tell friends and family about breast cancer)

Boss, C., & Boss, C. (2017). I have cancer, now what? 12 things you, your spouse, and your family must know in your battle with cancer. Sanger, CA: Familius LLC.

Inhestern, L., & Bergelt, C. (2018). When a mother has cancer: Strains and resources of affected families from the mother's and father's perspective – a qualitative study. BMC Women's Health, 18, 72. 10.1186/s12905-018-0562-8.

Lillie, H. M., Venetis, M. K., & Chernichky-Karcher, S. M. (2018). "He would never let me just give up": Communicatively constructing dyadic resilience in the experience of breast cancer. Health Communication, 33, 1516–1524. 10.1080/104100236.2017.1372049.

Magsamen-Conrad, K., Venetis, M. K., Checton, M. G., & Greene, K. (2019). The role of response perceptions in couples' ongoing cancer-related disclosure. Health Communication, 34, 999–1009. 10.1080/10410236.2018.1452091.

Weber, K. M., & Solomon, D. H. (2008). Locating relationship and communication issues among stressors associated with breast cancer. Health Communication, 23, 548–559. 10.1080/10410230802465233.

Reference

Fitzgerald, K., Paravati, E., Green, M. C., Moore, M. M., & Qian, J. L. (2020). Restorative narratives for health promotion. *Health Communication*, *35*, 356–363. 10.1080/10410236.2018.1563032.

12 Supporting the Children, and Children as Support

Women facing breast cancer who are living in a family with children of all ages, from the very young to older teens, have frequently reported the impact on their children is one of their added concerns. To mitigate such worries, this chapter discusses three principles. First we explain the likely psychological needs of any non-adult children in the immediate family. Next we suggest ways to address these needs, especially distress for their mother's health and appearance, fears of abandonment, and major changes in their life circumstances. Third, we consider how children and young people can be guided and encouraged to be supportive of her and especially helpful to you as primary caregiver.

We discuss children's knowledge of and feelings about breast cancer, including the possible distortions of information and magical ideas they might have. We offer strategies for children to use for coping with negative feelings. Their experiences need not be entirely negative, as new situations create opportunities to learn and express feelings of empathy for others. To ensure children's lives are disrupted as little as possible, we give ideas around creating household routines, establishing equitable expectations, and ensuring continued high levels of reward for cooperation and making some sacrifices. The chapter ends with an emphasis on family collaborative problem solving, using structured family meetings focused on establishing agreements and fairness for everyone in the family.

The wide divergence of family structures, family dynamics, and lifestyles, as well as the ages of mothers with breast cancer and the ages of her children, all make it difficult to lay down a firm set of do's and don'ts. So in this chapter we have tried not to give rigid directions but to explain what the route might look like, where the potholes might be, and which detours and shortcuts you might be able to take to navigate the inevitable challenges. As always we encourage such navigation to be worked out and conducted in collaboration with the mother – the woman you are caring for.

DOI: 10.4324/9781003194088-12

Families

We are defining *families* broadly: we include stepfamilies (a blend that's sometimes complicated in its own right) and families where there are two women or two men in parental roles. We're also including what are generally known as "extended families," in which the primary mothering role might be carried out partially or totally by a grandmother, aunt, adult sister, or foster mother – any one of whom might be susceptible to breast cancer.

You know grown-ups worry about our children, but children worry too. So we will explain how children can be a strength to you, and how they, with your help, can be concerned but not fearful. Our focus is on the dependent children, from toddlers to teenagers, who are living at home. Children in such families must cope with an array of significant challenges, including increased household responsibilities and inevitable changes in schedules. Worse, they may have to cope with her absences and even the threat of her dying.

Many research studies have confirmed a mother's breast cancer significantly increases stress levels in the children. Researchers have often found they are likely to experience anxiety and depression, as well as signs of stress such as headaches, avoiding social activities, oppositional behaviors, being irritable, or having difficulty sleeping. You may see an increase in bickering between siblings, being argumentative, seeking more attention, and getting lower grades at school. If some of these difficulties escalate it might be helpful to get a school counselor involved. But such gloomy outcomes are by no means inevitable, and there are ways of reducing the risks and preventing them from escalating into more serious emotional problems.

Mothers themselves will be aware of these risks. That has often been found in research studies. In one report, a psychologist in Portugal reviewed many such studies and confirmed that all over the world mothers with breast cancer felt particularly responsible for meeting their children's emotional and physical needs. They also tended to prioritize these needs in decision-making. A primary concern was whether they would be able to fulfill their maternal role and meet their responsibilities as a mother. You, therefore, might try to remember nothing of what we suggest as family adaptations for your children should result in undermining the woman's role as a good mother to her children.

Six Basic Principles for Families

Maternal breast cancer represents both the obvious and the more subtle challenges for the whole family. What we emphasize are positive and practical steps to answer questions you may have. What part can and should the children themselves play? How different should your expectations be depending on the children's ages, gender, and maturity? One key question related to children was addressed in the previous chapter: how and when do you best disclose the discovery that their mother has a serious illness? Chapter 11 covers those issues of privacy, disclosure, and sharing information with and by children. It is the first stage in your campaign to support the whole family and enlist their support for their mother and you.

There are six underlying truths we know from our experience and from numerous studies in scholarly journals that are especially relevant to the goals of this chapter:

- Once they know about the diagnosis, children will have ongoing fears, often undisclosed, both for their mother and for themselves. They may not talk about their worries, which is unfortunate as avoidance of negative emotional experiences often makes them worse.
- A child's ability to understand all that's going on will depend on their age, interests, and comfort with abstract ideas. Positive strategies need to be tailored to these individual differences in kids.
- Children's ability to show empathy and to rise to the occasion of another person's needs, particularly those of a loved one, is usually an established element of their personality. Empathy can have a downside, however: children's feelings of sorrow and distress for their mother can be so extreme they add to their own stress and thus to that of the family.
- How well children manage their stress and cope with challenges will determine the extent to which they can be counted on to be helpful and supportive. For you, therefore, enhancing their resilience (see Chapter 11) by fostering good coping strategies is yet another task to add to your to-do list.
- In a family, what affects one member affects all the others. Everyone is a working part of the whole, yet few families function like a well-oiled machine. Important components such as the strength of the family's emotional bonds ("cohesion"), the clarity of communication, and willingness to manage conflicts constructively, are parts sometimes a little rusty or worn down. Fortunately, however, this chapter is not about the perfect family; it is about the *good enough family* whose working parts might benefit from just a drop of oil here and there.
- In addition to recognizing possible changes in family roles, it is important to remember these will not be permanent. The children's

mother will recover; conditions will eventually return to a prior level of normality. While there may be some changes in the new normal, try to ensure the woman's role as a mother has not been undermined.

Children's Feelings About Breast Cancer

In order to understand the range and complexity of children's feelings, it is worth remembering emotions are partially related to the thoughts and ideas you and their mother have about any situation. Thus children's knowledge of breast cancer, and the words they hear and use to describe it, will influence how they feel about it.

Children's pre-existing ideas about cancer are likely to be quite different from yours. Younger children, for example, tend to use "magical thinking." Their magical beliefs about the world mean they can have really outlandish but widespread ideas about illness and treatments, not just the Tooth Fairy and monsters in the closet. Working with young children (5- to 6-year-olds) we have found there is a need to reassure them they won't catch others' chronic illnesses, or when someone gets an injection the needle won't poke out the other side. Many children have more general fears, such as panic at the sight of blood, or they may not like the physical atmosphere and smell of hospitals.

As soon as you and she have together told the children about their mother's cancer (see Chapter 11) ask them what they know about cancer. Whether their thoughts and beliefs are truly rational and appropriate can easily be judged by asking further questions and listening to the answers rather than simply telling them things. If they have fantastical or magical ideas you can gently give them reassurance and more accurate information. Generally you and their mother can do this together, but there may be ideas and concerns they want to share with you rather than upset her with too many questions

No matter how much the children respect your knowledge, children will have gleaned information from movies, friends, social media, and school. A team of nursing and psychology researchers from China and Australia studied children's understanding of breast cancer. All the children, regardless of age, knew cancer was a scary, sometimes fatal disease. "Some cancers can't be cured" one child said. One 9-year-old girl described, "a malignant tumor is a kind of tumor having a vicious circle, and the cancer cells can transfer from one place to another. Actually I can't explain it clearly ... A cancer cell is a kind of fatal cell." All of the children knew the name and concept of chemotherapy. They knew it was a cause of hair loss – one boy said he had learned it in biology class at school. But they were also aware that hair loss would be only temporary–one child said she knew it because her grandmother had reassured her of that. They also reported mothers would be tired and "throw up a lot" as a result of chemotherapy. The authors of this study concluded that most of the children's perceptions were relatively realistic, but the details were not always accurate.

But a little knowledge, even if largely correct, can be a dangerous thing. So the first step to managing children's emotions is to ensure they are based on clear thinking. But that may not be sufficient since understanding rarely dispels negative emotions arising from the way we judge situations as threatening or dangerous. When a child is confronted with the reality that his or her mother has a serious medical condition requiring hospitalization, the first emotion experienced will be fear. The most basic fear is their mother might die. Fear of being abandoned is primal, especially in the youngest children.

The next fear is they might somehow catch it. This second fear will really only be present in younger children. But remember our discussion of genetic counseling (p. 171). Older children, especially girls, could well have feelings of alarm they themselves may have breast cancer one day. In a careful research project in which 140 children across six US states were interviewed, the one dread linking all the children's concerns together was "losing her." This included the mother being away in hospital, that she might die, thinking about her being sick and in surgery, seeing the mother as physically and emotionally changed, and "mom not being able to take care of me."

A third fear children have reported is more subtle. When the illness is breast cancer, many children will know mastectomy is a likely possible treatment, raising fears of disfigurement for their mother and also possibly longer-term implications of being less able to do everyday things in the future. And as breasts are sexual objects somewhat taboo for younger boys, there is likely to be embarrassment in discussing them.

A fourth fear blends into sorrow and worry about what all this will mean for their mother. Without wanting to recognize it in themselves, there may be nagging worries about how the situation might disrupt their own plans and sources of well-being. That is perfectly natural and cannot be attributed to selfishness and self-interest – children have a right as well as a need to expect their parents to provide a level of stability, now and in the future. The children's emotional relationship, their bond, with their mother will be different from their relationship with you. So you won't be able to be a perfect substitute. Try to allow time for simple contact with their mother.

To put all this together, most children in the family of a woman with breast cancer will experience a degree of initial distress, not always expressed in words. In younger children, for example, you may see a sudden increase in bed-wetting. In slightly older children, stomach pains and headaches, temper tantrums, and angrily answering back are all signs of confused feelings. As a result, it would be useful for you to be alert to possible changes in their everyday behavior, and you may need to cut them some slack as your children try to cope with a situation over which they have no control and makes them feel helpless. That means showing patience, tolerance, pausing before you criticize and then saying something that shows you might be feeling the same way they are. In a later section we describe how admitting and labeling your own feelings is a teaching moment that helps children better understand their own.

Coping with Negative Feelings (and Boosting Constructive Ones)

In this next section we explain how children themselves try to deal with negative emotions – their *coping strategies*. How they cope influences how stress will impact them and whether it causes further disruptive behavior. Everyone experiences stress in life but knowing how to cope with negative feelings and solve challenges and problems determines their degree of *resilience*.

If you look up "children's coping strategies" on the Internet, you will find literally thousands of articles. We will describe just one widely accepted model which organizes all the different ways of coping into four main types: problem-focused, emotion-focused, support-seeking, and meaning-making coping.

- *Problem-focused* strategies are largely what this book is all about. These strategies involve the child dealing actively with the source of the stress, such as getting more accurate information, or learning new skills to help manage a problem. This includes things like children needing to learn more about breast cancer or rolling up their sleeves and doing things to be really helpful for the mother.
- *Emotion-focused* strategies include things like releasing pent up emotions. Being allowed to have a really good cry can be positive but lashing out with anger is not very helpful. Any direct attempts by the child to control or manage their feelings fit into this category, for example, avoidance or denial (not thinking about the implications of the cancer for their mother) and distraction (thinking of other, more pleasant things). It is a coping strategy if your child

looks for any positive aspect of what has happened, such as being able to recognize occasional humorous elements. You, along with their mother, can assist your kids in using this "glass is half-full" strategy by emphasizing aspects like the cancer was caught early, the doctors are very well trained, and everyone is pulling together so our family will end up stronger as a result.

- *Social support seeking* strategies are generally very helpful and should be encouraged in conjunction with any others. Support from friends and extended family members comes in many forms. Some of it is simply *practical* – a friend's mom or dad might volunteer to drive your youngster to softball practice. Encourage him or her to accept gracefully. We also all need our friends and family to *reassure* us, to have someone to talk to, someone to whom we can confess our worst fears and nightmares.

  The only drawback is that some of your children's friends or family members, in trying to be helpful, may be less skilled at listening and suggesting problem-solving solutions. They may instead inadvertently exacerbate negative feelings. So try to discover what a friend's response was, so you can judge its helpfulness. The value of other children's replies like the following can be judged with a little common sense: "OMG, how dreadful for your mom. I'm so sorry for you. I had an aunt who died of breast cancer"; "Wow that sucks – you're going to have to look after your two little brothers a lot more"; "Keep talking to me. Call or text me any time you feel down. I'm here for you. Give your mom my love." It's usually easy to recognize good social support. So, it would generally be helpful for you to encourage your children to talk about their concerns with their friends but also encourage them to share what they hear. Be sure to remind them about the importance of respecting their mother's wishes for privacy and appropriate disclosures (p. 167–170, Chapter 11).

- *Meaning-making coping* is the fourth strategy commonly identified by psychologists. It describes how we as humans try to deal with tragic events by attributing some sort of meaning to them. It is also the most controversial coping strategy because it depends heavily on your family values, religious beliefs, and culture. For example, Swedish people tend to use meditation when thinking about the meaning of cancer; Korean people reported using prayer, and faith in healthy eating; Turkish families facing cancer focused on existential thoughts of their inner strength and about the meaning of family love. Even if your family has a strong religious faith, there are large differences between thinking of some misfortune as God's punishment and seeing illness and tragedy as part of God's plan. If you and your children seek solace from a minister of religion one would hope the focus is on cherishing what you have that is good and can be thankful for and finding purpose from your family's love for each other.

Ideally too, meaning-making coping refers neither to denial of their mother's cancer nor to excessive over-reaction emotionally, but to relating the illness to meaningful things in the child's life. So try to avoid words that catastrophize and blame, like "victim," "disaster," "tragedy," "God's angry." In professional counseling there is a great deal of current interest in the idea of *acceptance* – finding peace with the way things are rather than wishing they were otherwise. Your children may hear their mother apologizing for the trouble she is causing and for being such a burden. You can help them have ready answers to say to her if this happens: "no one is to blame"; "we're all going to deal with it"; "our family is a circle of strength," "Dad's given us stuff to read about what causes cancer" – whatever sounds right to you.

Recognizing these four types of coping is useful, but most children use more than one style of coping. They often use a variety of different strategies, some of which may work quite well in the short-term. A Norwegian interview study of young children living with a parent with cancer found they were able to cope and have good quality of life by switching in and out from one strategy to another. Regardless of your children's coping styles it is easy to see how a close family could get caught up in too much open discussion and focus on everybody's worries and needs and general mental health. The best type of coping is for the family to focus on solutions rather than the problems.

Children's Empathy

It may sound absurd to say there is ever an upside to serious illness in a family. However, our clinical experience confirms that children like to be useful and want to help, so many families are able to find strengths from the experience of coping with adversity. Clear positives such as changed family priorities, taking pleasure in a mother's recovery, greater appreciation of life, and increased faith and spirituality, have been reported by families. Especially valuable benefits arise when you and the children increase your ability to understand, accept, and prioritize the needs and experiences of another person. This fosters children's *empathy,* which increases family cohesion and helps children support their mother and you during a difficult time.

From a very young age (as early as 2) most children are able to show empathy – understanding and concern for the feelings of others, and putting themselves in others' shoes. There can also be reasons why feelings of concern for others might not be strong in some children. For example, certain disabilities such as autism make it much harder for children to understand their own feelings, much less the feelings of others.

If you sense your child has difficulty in expressing empathy for their mother and cannot understand fully what she might be going through, there are opportunities to teach a few simple *emotion competencies*. That is the phrase child psychologists use for the ability to understand and label one's own feelings and to recognize the feelings of others from the situation, their facial expression, and the most obvious signs of emotion such as smiling or crying.

We also want to make sure the child understands sympathy is not quite the same as empathy. In fact for someone with breast cancer, expressions of sympathy might be quite aversive and counterproductive. The only way sympathy can be encouraged is if it leads to determined action to improve matters. Saying lines like "my thoughts and prayers are with you" is less meaningful if you are not doing anything to alleviate the hurt or harm someone has experienced.

There are a few easily adopted ideas to help children gain emotion competence:

• *Help them label feelings, starting with your own, when an everyday situation calls for it:* "I felt quite *scared* when I heard car tires screeching outside. When I went out to investigate I was *relieved* to see that no-one was hurt. It *annoys* me when people drive so fast down our road they have to slam on their brakes when the traffic light turns red. I'm *happy* all our neighbors are petitioning for speed bumps on our street. That gives me *hope* we'll get people to *feel more responsible* for kids playing in this street, and slow down."

• *Your own and others' feelings can be identified and labeled:* "I cheered when you scored that goal at the soccer game! It made your mom and me *happy*. We were really *proud* of you because I know how hard you have been practicing. I'm sure the other team's goalie was *disappointed*, but they should be *delighted* at how many other goal kicks they saved."

The point of these slightly artificial examples of emotion talk is that in almost any conversation, words can be introduced to elaborate on complex feelings. It shows you have them, and helps your child recognize feelings that may explain otherwise uncharacteristic behavior.

If you follow this logic through you will see your disclosure of your own feelings about the person you are caring for is in itself an *emotion learning opportunity* for your children Acknowledging you are worried about her – and are even sad at times – will represent an authentic expression of an emotion. This is far more helpful to children of all ages than trying to always put a brave face on things (pretending you are not scared) and minimize your feelings of concern. After you have expressed honest negative feelings, however, you can then model an appropriate coping thought or strategy:

- "I am scared, but I really trust mom's doctors" or "but I have faith in the Lord."
- "I think before we get too worried we need to think of something constructive we can do for mom. Let's ask her what would be helpful."
- "Everyone's feeling so sad now, why don't you talk with mom about something pleasant or cheerful.

Disruption to Children's Lives and Establishing Household Routines

Canadian professor of nursing Ann Hilton and her colleagues (see Sources for More Information at the end of this chapter) studied the perspectives of men coping with their wives' breast cancer. They quoted one dad as saying: "*When mom's sick things grind to a halt. It's macaroni and wieners.*" It's an amusing example of something many of us have experienced, but there is a serious side to the comment. It cleverly illustrates the issues in this section of the chapter: how your role in the family might change; how to make sure everyday life and standards don't deteriorate; and how children can pitch in and help around the house (after all, any teenager can put together macaroni and wieners and probably something much better for dinner!)

Our basic advice is that all the kids in the family can be hugely supportive to the mother with breast cancer and to you – the primary adult partner. There is a caveat we need to mention. While men who have been interviewed about their perspectives on coping with breast cancer have often said things like "I've become the mom now," it's important to remember there are lots of things the real mom will still be able to do for the children. And she will want to still do these things, so you have to let her, without fussing. In other words, make sure the children in their eagerness to help don't turn their mother into a powerless patient. It won't make her better to feel she is being easily replaced! Children should not take on a nursing role or be her personal helper. The best policy is always to ask her what would be helpful and to remember what would be helpful to her can change over time.

When children's help is clearly needed and appropriate it can be active and constructive, or passive and tolerant. Active help means taking on new responsibilities, helping with food preparation, folding the laundry, taking out the trash, mowing the lawn, walking the dog – indeed all the sorts of chores many families require of their children from time to time. With a seriously ill person in the house, however, it is important that these chores be done regularly, willingly, and without argument – well, reminders and asking a second time is okay, and realistic!

Passive help means children not doing things they might otherwise do. To help you out with chores you may find yourself doing, they could be encouraged not to throw into the laundry basket clothes they've only worn once! Helping by not doing could extend to not insisting on watching a particular TV show the mother hates, using earphones to listen to one's favorite music or when playing video games, and possibly giving up activities requiring transportation or a great deal of adult supervision time, which will be in short supply. Children will have to make sacrifices, perhaps doubling up in bedrooms so the mother can have a bedroom to herself for a few weeks, or not having friends over for a wild birthday party. And as you may be facing major increases in medical bills, they will need to be reminded that expensive activities previously taken for granted, may be on hold for a while. "Next year, honey" is a useful phrase – but really mean it!

Here is the key to all this. You will know children are acutely aware of personal justice and fairness. If you haven't heard your children from age about 4 to 18 say "But that's not FAIR!" then you don't have children! Children remember when an older sibling was first allowed to use make-up, who got to ride in the front seat on the last big outing three years ago, who was allowed to ride their bike to school and at what age, and who got the last scoop of ice-cream last weekend. Children as young as five can judge the fairness of a situation on the basis of principles of social justice and can show empathy for the feelings of other children who have been left out or wrongly blamed. So remember this one cardinal principle: everything that happens within the family should be equitable. That doesn't mean treating everyone exactly the same: there will be differences based on ages, abilities, and specific levels of responsibility. What it does mean is that if sacrifices are required and previous privileges and rewards are lost under the new crisis conditions, they must be shared evenhandedly by the family.

Given that children differ in abilities, the key to fairness is to devise activities, rewards, or opportunities that are the approximate equivalent of those assigned to any one sibling. If one child has to do certain tasks or achieve specified grades at school in order to get a reward, an equivalent reward needs to be available for another child doing a similar task. In some of our research on children's perception of fairness, we soon learned if you want to find out what children consider fair, just ask them! There is simply no point trying to argue higher ideals, like playing the maturity card: "You're old enough and responsible enough to give up your bedroom for a few weeks," without some fair compensation.

We think this issue is so much common sense we're not going to give lots of examples. But we recommend that any new household procedure requiring some degree of extra work by a child, or some loss of a previous pleasure, has to be agreed upon by all – a family discussion in which you say: "Everything is negotiable – it just has to be *fair* to everyone in this family. Remember what happened to mom, and what she is going through is definitely not fair. So think about how we are going to manage as a family with everyone taking their fair share of what needs to be done. Just because you're older – or younger, or you're a girl/boy, or you're the kid I always rely on, or you're so good at helping out, or you're strong – we're actually all together in the same canoe, gang. So all of us are going to paddle together and in the same direction." We're not trying to put precise words in your mouth. These are examples and it's up to you how you wish to convey this critical principle.

There is one technique which will make fairness in your family pretty well guaranteed and reduce arguments and recriminations, and that is to set up formal routines. OK, maybe you are a free spirit, love chaos, enjoy a haphazard lifestyle, and have never insisted on rules or adherence to dates and times – we promise you, now is the time to change! You need to set up regular schedules everyone understands, accepts, and promises to follow. Make sure at least half of the things in the list are fun and enjoyable – one night can be pizza delivery night, Tuesday evenings can be soppy comedy movie night on TV, on Saturday's picnic in the park everyone makes their own sandwich. Predictability in life is one of the best ways to manage anxiety – uncertainty causes stress. And remember, if you don't like lists and charts on the fridge door, one of your children might be really good at setting up schedules on their computer and, if we're talking older teenagers, know how to send reminder text messages to everyone's cell phone. Knowing what is happening next and what things are coming up really helps shoving stress out the door.

But with a breast cancer patient in the house there are many things that might happen unexpectedly, so some of your routines might have to be flexible, with a substitute activity on hand. If mom is feeling repulsed by the smell of certain foods wafting through the house, try alternatives for the time being: pizza-with-anchovies night might be replaced by "Who can think of the healthiest salad?" or "What's the blandest chip dip we can mix up?"

The simplest way to maintain a routine is a good wall calendar in which activities and events are carefully written down; this allows everyone to know what is happening. This reduces conflict over reasonable changes if last-minute opportunities come up – a typical example might be one kid gets invited for a play date, but you had planned something else for that weekend.

Rewards and Sacrifices

It's easy to summarize our recommendations for the daily activities of your children in your family: keep things normal! As much as possible it is helpful for children if you can maintain as many of the same activities and routines that were typical before cancer threw a monkey-wrench into your household. All sorts of usual activities can be seriously disrupted. Maybe mom is the one who usually helps with homework, or she's the one who always used to drive your children to soccer practice or organized play dates and sleepovers with other parents.

If yours is a blended family, she may have been the one who arranges for the kids in the house to spend alternate weekends with their dad and takes over the swimsuit that's been forgotten. Change responsibilities around based on the nature of the activity and the timetable of treatment. Following surgery or chemo, chauffeuring may not be feasible, but mom may be perfectly capable of and want to make the phone calls. If one thing mom usually did has to go by the board, find an equivalent activity which can be done instead with other grown-ups. In the study Hilton and others carried out, where at least one child resided at home, a major theme was trying to keep patterns normal and family life going. As one father explained: "It's important to keep everything in perspective and continue to do simple things: watching the sunset, going for a walk, eating at our family's favorite restaurant, watching a great movie, doing stuff with their friends."

At the same time, however, as nothing will now be exactly the same as before, you might try seizing the opportunity to introduce new positive routines and activities that will strengthen family functioning. Start a new tradition: find an interesting new board game and designate the one evening per week everyone will gather round to play; teach your child to cook; redecorate a child's bedroom. We could make a long list of possibilities but select activities that feel comfortable to you and your family.

These two suggestions may seem like contradictions: always do the familiar, versus add something new. However, if you remember the goal is to foster the family atmosphere most likely to be helpful to you and the woman you're supporting, you can maintain a good balance between these two broad recommendations. Another way of thinking of this balance is in terms of rewards and sacrifices. The children in your family will all have to make some sacrifices – giving up space, favorite events, and time with one and more likely both of their parents. No matter how empathic and giving your child might be, these losses of fun times and meaningful experiences can lead to feelings of resentment. Loss of routine behaviors and their rewards, and loss of positive expectations for the future, are widely considered to be factors contributing to depression. To help balance these losses, ensuring as many opportunities for rewards as possible is the other half of the equation.

Everyone in the family unit will have to make some sacrifices. Many religious faiths see sacrifice as something that helps to develop a person's character. If this applies to your situation then by all means use such principles to give your child a sense of purpose behind what they might be having to give up. Many would argue sacrificing something for someone else or for your faith brings its own rewards. And if religion plays an important part in your life that might be the best way to pitch it to your children. Other families may not be at all religious but instead adhere to social and moral principles based on responsibility to care for others as well as oneself.

What we suggest is you aid such a process by consciously looking for ways of adding extra rewards – praise, special "quality time" (family activities done together that everyone enjoys), and even low-cost material rewards like small increases in pocket money, free public events and outings, trips to their favorite fast food restaurant. The children's mother may have some good ideas about possible rewards.

Rewards can be spontaneous (creating pleasant surprises, catching someone being good and acknowledging it), or they can be contingent on some agreed upon accomplishment. This is called *reinforcement* in psychology – there need to be positive consequences for desired behaviors. A simple way to formalize any such arrangement is through the idea of a contract. In some types of family therapy these contracts are quite detailed and written out and even signed by both the parent and the child or teenager. You don't have to go that far, but it can be quite fun to draw up a contract and decide what duties are being agreed upon and what the rewards for successful completion of a task will be. There are many examples of such contracts on the Internet – see the end of the chapter.

Bringing It All Together: The Family Conference

To state the obvious, families are complex. The *dynamics* (who controls, influences, decides, dominates) vary from family to family, culture to culture. Parenting style is often described by family psychologists as fitting somewhere along two dimensions. One is a *control* dimension, going from permissive (easy going) at one end, to strict (firm rules), at the opposite ends. The other dimension is *acceptance,* going from being very accepting (warm, sensitive, and loving) versus rejecting (colder, more austere). Psychologists have identified a parenting style that reduces conflict and fosters good family relationships and minimal problems as "authoritative" parenting. *Authoritative* (not "authoritarian") parenting is a style combining high levels on the sensitivity and warmth dimension, with a middle level on the control dimension by setting clear limits and consistent boundaries. Authoritative parents use reasoning and explanations to discipline their children, rewarding good behavior rather than relying on threats and punishments for bad behavior.

You may or may not see yourself in these descriptions, and this is not the time to tell you about every possible strategy of good parenting – remember, you only need to be good enough! There is, however, one very useful and very simple technique that *can* easily be adopted by any family. It might be called a family meeting, a family conference, or a problem-solving session. It works along the general principles of restorative justice – when dealing with any issue, at the end of the discussion all participants need to feel they have been respected, listened to, and heard. Good family conferences are quite formal affairs. They need to be planned with a designated time and place. In principle any member of the family can call one, but typically it will be the parents as heads of the household. The rules are simple, everyone gets a chance to speak and air their grievance or concerns. No one can shout at, or put down, accuse, or criticize anyone else. Whining is not allowed! The purpose is to generate a solution to whatever issue is raised and the solution must be agreed by everyone present and judged as fair. A family collaborative problem-solving process requires exactly the same steps as would be used in business meetings or in the management of any agency. These are illustrated in Box 12.1.

Every family has a set of rules and expectations. Sometimes children break these rules, which can be a perfectly natural source of conflict within families. Now, however, you are faced with an entirely new set of conditions. Mom is recuperating from surgery at home. She may not be in pain, but she may be extremely uncomfortable. She is undergoing treatment which makes her feel lousy. New rules need to be set and they

---

Box 12.1   Five Steps for Family Collaborative Problem Solving

1. *Identify the issue:* "What's happening here?" To identify the issue, state the desired outcome. Avoid referring to the issue as a problem.
2. *Generate all possible solutions:* "What can we do?" Brainstorm potential solutions. Don't limit creativity – discuss all suggestions without any value judgments. You want to identify possible alternatives to what is currently happening.
3. *Screen solutions for feasibility:* "What would really work?" Once all the solutions have been suggested, review each one in light of the following criteria:
4. Does it represent this family's values?
5. Is the solution feasible – can we implement it, do we have time, do we have the materials, can we afford it?
6. Predict the possible outcomes of each solution – what are the pros and cons?
7. *Choose the solution to implement:* "Let's take action!" All members of the family must express consensus on which solution to implement; this helps ensure support for and commitment to the solution by everyone.
8. *Evaluate the solution implemented:* "How did we do? Did it work? What changed?" Everyone needs to be asked whether your family plan had its intended effect. Was the issue resolved? Did everyone get what they needed? How are you feeling about it now? Do we need to go back to the drawing board?

---

are based on the needs of just one person, whose preferences and desires must take precedence, at least for the time being. If you can introduce new rules based on caring principles and your family's values, as well as on the health and safety of the mother, they will all be accepted just as long as you try to also respect the personal rights and freedoms of the children. This reasoning can be explained and discussed in a family group conference. This helps the children in the family accept some restrictions of their personal liberties when the goal is to help maintain family harmony and their mother's progress towards recovery.

It's fascinating to think a little about the future – a child's perception of time is so different from an adult's. Imagine when their mother might be judged free of all cancer, perhaps at her five-year checkup. That would be a moment to look forward to and celebrate. But think of what that time span means for your children. In five years' time your child who just started middle school when their mother was first diagnosed might now be graduating from high school. In five years an older teen in your family might have learned a trade and been working for three years, even married and with a baby so you and she are now a grandparents! Other kids might be going to college, finishing grade school, gone overseas, or have bought a house in another state – all major transitions. Organize a family group conference to think about life five or seven years from now and how you all together will celebrate the news their mother's oncologist no longer needs to see her annually – or ever again. This helps create realistic expectations for the future that are not guaranteed but place the focus on the continuity of life and how dramatically time moves forward for children compared to yours.

Summary and Recommendations

- There is no need for a family situation to "become chaotic." The key thing about remembering to *plan and stick to family routines* is that as much as possible for children we want their lives to be similar, in practical terms, to the way they were before their mother's illness.
- In being supported and *being supportive*, children's own emotional development can be boosted, and their resilience increased.
- Recognize the likely *complexity of your children's feelings*, and openly acknowledge and explain your own.
- Help your children *understand accurate information* about the nature of breast cancer to minimize any false information or fanciful ideas they might have.
- Organize your family as a *team* devoted to making everything as smooth and as easy as possible for their mother, while being sensitive to their mom's preferences.
- Recognize the *importance of fostering empathy* in the children, but ensure if sacrifices have to be made, principles of *fairness* are adhered to.
- *Reward* the activities you want the children to participate in and express warm and unconditional *positive feelings* for each other (family cohesion),

- Establish clear *boundaries with consistent routines* to keep stability in the family while maximizing rewards, both social and material.
- Encourage different *strategies for coping with negative feelings* and formal family group meetings to work through any problems. Use a *collaborative problem-solving strategy*, which will require the collaboration and ideas from every family member as an equal participant.
- These are all aspirations worth working towards for the health of the whole family and the woman with breast cancer. *There is no one way which is the only correct way*, but if the general principles are clear in your mind, these elements will all fall into place, not perfectly, but close enough.

Sources for More Information

https://www.huffpost.com/entry/childrens-books-about-cancer_l_5e32f5 efc5b611ac94d0e347 (a list of 15 books written for children about cancer that you might find useful, but check their descriptions first to see if you like the sound of them, as we are not endorsing any of them individually)

https://breastcancernow.org/information-support/facing-breast-cancer/talking-children-about-breast-cancer (discusses how to talk to children of different ages about breast cancer)

https://www.pinterest.com/acnlatitudes/behavior-contracts-printables/ (offers examples of *contracts* between parent and child)

Almulla, H. A., & Lewis, F. M. (2020). Losing her: Children's reported concerns in the first 6 months of their mother's breast cancer diagnosis. Cancer Nursing, 43, 514–520.

Hilton, B. A., Crawford, J. A., & Tarko, M. A. (2000). Men's - perspectives on individual and family coping with their wives' breast cancer and chemotherapy. Western Journal of Nursing Research, 22, 438–459.

Huang, X., O'Connor, M., Hu, Y, Gao, H., & Lee, S. (2018). Children's understanding of maternal breast cancer: A qualitative study. European Journal of Oncology Nursing, 34, 8–14.

Tavares, R., Brandão, T., & Matos, P. M. (2018). Mothers with breast cancer: A mixed-method systematic review on the impact on the parent-child relationship. Psycho-Oncology, 27, 367–375.

13 Metastatic Breast Cancer and End-of-Life

This chapter addresses the worst-case scenario: her breast cancer is not cured. Her doctors have advised that she has advanced cancer and will need treatment for the remainder of her life. Unlike earlier stage breast cancer, Stage IV or Metastatic Breast Cancer (MBC) does not involve choosing time-limited treatments to achieve a normal, cancer-free future. Instead, she will make decisions about ongoing treatments – one after the other – intended to limit the spread and manage the symptoms of MBC. These decisions can buy more time and affect her quality of life, so she must weigh the relative benefits versus side effects of different treatments. She may decide a treatment is making her so much sicker that the reduction of her quality of life and ability to do normal things is no longer worth the promise of more months of a life she considers unacceptably compromised. Once breast cancer has spread to other organs and parts of the body, there is no way to avoid facing uncomfortable and painful discussions and decisions. Because MBC could become your reality, our book would not be honest had we ignored this possibility and not included this chapter.

Not all breast cancers will be cured, but science is pushing the boundaries of what we know about effective treatment and care even as you are reading this page. She may have an opportunity to participate in a research clinical trial to improve her condition and perhaps even lead to a major break-through. Nor is the diagnosis an immediate death sentence: At the time of this writing, women with MBC are living an average of 2–3 years beyond that diagnosis – and many survive for five years or more. As a young mother living with MBC, Adiba Barney (see Sources For More Information at the end of this chapter) published a candid and uplifting book about her experiences since her initial breast cancer diagnosis in her twenties: she shares her hopes and fears, but never loses her focus on confronting what she knows to be her final years in a way that makes "margaritas" out of the "cactuses" thrust her way.

DOI: 10.4324/9781003194088-13

No matter what her age or how many years are likely to remain of her life, you will want to support her during this final and most challenging time of all. Imagine, too, how much additional years with a good quality of life could mean to her, giving her a time for watching and being there for her children and others whom she loves – including you. Everyone will want those remaining times to be the best that they can be. You and she will not want those years to be shrouded in dread and overwhelmed by suffering, overshadowing happier memories in her life. This can be a time for her to control her legacy even if she cannot control the cancer. This chapter is about supporting her no matter what.

What Is Metastatic Breast Cancer?

Approximately 20–30% of women diagnosed with an earlier stage breast cancer (Stages 0–III) later develop MBC; this is in addition to the 6% who already had metastatic disease at the first diagnosis of breast cancer (diagnosed as "de novo metastatic"). This is called Stage IV cancer in the U.S. and many other countries and called Secondary Cancer in other countries such as the UK. At earlier stages, additional tumors may signal recurrences of the primary breast cancer or simply that another disease site has been identified. But Stage IV is different: the cancer is no longer restricted to the breasts and nearby lymph nodes but has traveled elsewhere in the body through the bloodstream or lymphatic system.

In MBC/Stage IV/Secondary Cancer, the original (Primary) breast cancer has spread to other organs or parts of the body. Most often, these Secondary Cancers first appear in the brain, liver, lungs, or bones such as the ribs, spine, pelvis, or the long bones in arms and legs. These additional cancers in other locations in the body are also breast cancer because the cancer cells are the same type as those originally diagnosed in the breast. They are not a second cancer or a new cancer that could develop (unrelated to breast cancer) later in life. For example, breast cancer cells metastasized to the lungs are not the same as lung cancer, and her doctor's treatment will reflect this.

Box 13.1 lists the most common sites for the spread of breast cancer and likely symptoms, so you and she can monitor for any signs of metastasis. If she is experiencing any of the symptoms listed in Box 13.1, support her to contact her doctor right away.

The diagnosis of MBC is never good news. It means your loved one is unlikely to survive and live the long life she originally envisioned. Her future days will entail ongoing treatment to prolong life and control symptoms and side effects. Nevertheless, this diagnosis should not mean giving up. From 2007 to 2017, overall cancer death rates decreased by

---

Box 13.1 Locations and Signs of Metastatic Breast Cancer

- *Bone:* Over half of MBC cases begin with spread to bones, causing a sudden, new pain that comes and goes at first but then becomes constant. This could be in the ribs, spine, pelvis, or the long bones in the arms or legs.

- *Lung:* MBC to the lungs could involve pain, discomfort, shortness of breath, a persistent cough lasting more than 1–2 weeks, wheezing, and coughing up blood or mucus. Often there are no symptoms.

- *Brain:* Spread to the brain can cause headaches, slurred speech, vision problems, dizziness and loss of balance, memory problems, mood/personality changes, and even seizures. The risk for spread to the brain is highest for HER2-positive or triple-negative cancers.

- *Liver:* There may be no symptoms when *mets* (breast cancer metastasized tumors) have spread to the liver. If there are symptoms, they include pain or discomfort in the mid-section, weakness and fatigue, a poor appetite and unexplained weight loss, fever, bloating, leg swelling, and a yellow tint to the skin or whites of the eyes.

15% due to many factors. Even though MBC is considered incurable, Stage IV cancers can be treated to extend life and manage symptoms for a good quality of life – many years into the future for more and more women. Nevertheless, at some point, Stage IV cancer will be considered terminal. Hence, we include planning for the time when you and she may be given this final prognosis.

Treatment Choices

Treatments for MBC are largely variations of those already described for earlier stage breast cancer. The major groups of systemic therapy for MBC are chemotherapy, hormonal/endocrine therapy, targeted drug therapies, and immunotherapies. The treatments available for her MBC will depend upon the type of breast cancer she has, where her cancer has metastasized, her overall health, and any other medical conditions. Recommendations for treatment may change from year to year as new treatments become available from advances in medical research (see the next section on clinical trials). Because she will need treatment for the rest of her life, her oncologist will also plan regular treatment "breaks" with her to allow relief from uncomfortable side effects. An excellent source for up-to-date information on current treatments for Stage IV breast cancer can be found on the American Cancer Society's website at: https://www.cancer.org/cancer/breast-cancer/treatment/treatment-of-breast-cancer-by-stage/treatment-of-stage-iv-advanced-breast-cancer.html. You and she can also click on a link at this site to "Chat with an Expert."

We are not going to provide a comprehensive list of possible treatments here or name specific targeted therapies. That would be a disservice to our readers: any list would quickly become outdated with new discoveries. Instead, this section presents summary information regarding currently available treatment choices for different breast cancer types and locations of the spread of MBC. These may be prescribed to attack the cancer itself and/or to relieve cancer symptoms depending on where the metastasized cancer tumors are located. By being informed about these treatments and their side effects, you will be in a better position to support her.

Systemic Drug Treatments

Systemic drugs are a main treatment for MBC, as they are for earlier stages of breast cancers (see Chapters 2 and 7). The types of drugs prescribed for advanced cancer will be based on the hormone receptor status and the HER2 status of the cancer (see Chapter 7). These treatments may continue – with possible treatment "breaks" – for weeks, months, or even years. A specific treatment will be continued until the cancer grows again or side effects become intolerable. When that happens, her oncologist typically recommends another drug based, again, on her specific cancer type and location of the spread. Major drug treatments including combinations for advanced Stage IV breast cancer include:

- *Chemotherapy*: Chemotherapy is often the first treatment for women with MBC and is especially recommended for MBC with triple-negative or HER2+ disease. Hormone therapy may be preferred but can take months to work against the cancer, so chemo may be prescribed first if she is extremely ill (i.e., her organs are shutting down). Chemotherapy is also the treatment of choice for women with hormone receptor-negative cancers (ER-negative and PR-negative, see Chapter 2, p. 20); hormone therapy is not effective with these cancers.

- *Hormone Therapy*: Treatment for women with hormone receptor-positive cancers may initially involve hormone therapy (tamoxifen or an aromatase inhibitor), perhaps combined with another targeted inhibitor drug. For HER2-positive cancers, Herceptin can help her live longer when used alongside chemotherapy, hormone therapy, or other anti-HER2 drugs. If she has a BRCA mutation, cancer drugs referred to as PARP inhibitors are prescribed.

- *Targeted Therapies and Immunotherapy Drugs*: Targeted therapies attack specific characteristics of cancer cells, such as the protein responsible for rapid or abnormal growth of cancer cells. These drugs are less likely than chemotherapy to harm healthy, non-cancerous cells. The most common form of MBC is ER+/HER2- which is typically treated with a combination of hormonal and targeted therapies. For triple-negative MBC when the woman has what is called a PDL-1 expressing cancer, an immunotherapy drug combined with chemotherapy is likely. Immunotherapy works by allowing her own immune system to attack the cancer more effectively.

As we discuss below and in previous chapters, the side effects, impact on her day-to-day quality of life, and needs for support will vary across different systemic treatments.

Local or Regional Treatments

Local and regional treatments such as surgery, radiation, or regional chemotherapy are also used to treat Stage IV cancers, often in conjunction with systemic drugs. These treatments are prescribed to manage symptoms, prevent complications, and provide pain relief rather than to cure the cancer. For example, a high percentage of MBC involves spread to the weight-bearing spine and hip bones and the long bones of the arms and legs, causing fractures. Treatment for a bone tumor may reduce the risk of fractures, not eliminate the cancer. Bone metastases may be also treated with radiation or bone-modifying agents such as bisphosphonates or denosumab to manage pain and reduce the risk of fractures. Here are other examples where surgery and/or radiation interventions may be prescribed primarily to help alleviate symptoms and prevent complications:

- *Brain*: whole brain radiation therapy or gamma knife radiation therapy may be used.
- *Liver*: a blood vessel can be unblocked using local therapies such as microwave ablation, radiofrequency ablation, and targeted anti-cancer drugs.

- *Bone*: a tumor is targeted to control pain, reduce the risk of fractures, or release pressure on the spinal cord.
- *Lungs*: breathing difficulties can be relieved.
- *Breast tumor*: radiation and/or surgery can tackle a tumor that is causing an open wound in the chest.

Be sure you and she clarify with her doctor whether a treatment is intended to try to cure the cancer or to manage symptoms. This may become particularly relevant two or more years following her diagnosis of MBC, when a cure is less likely and treatments may be interfering with other priorities in her life. Clarifying the main purpose of a treatment will help her decide whether and when to continue with treatments causing negative side effects that disrupt what she prefers to do with her remaining time. Women with young children at home may have a different approach to these issues compared with someone older who need not worry about her children growing up without her.

Participation in Clinical Trials

Cancer research is ongoing in hundreds of medical centers and research laboratories across the U.S. and around the world. Clinical trials of new, experimental treatments are being conducted all the time in medical research hospitals and facilities – some near you. These clinical trials follow established research protocols to test whether new therapies and treatments are effective. Medications are not approved for general use until they have been through rigorous scientific experimentation, so access to experimental treatments is only possible through voluntary participation in a clinical trial. For example, a particular clinical trial may be focused on a new drug developed to shrink existing tumors in a particular organ or part of the body. To investigate whether the new drug works, researchers test it on volunteers diagnosed with the exact cancer type and stage for which the medication is intended. Each drug will focus on a particular aspect of cancer – prevention, screening, treatment, supportive and palliative care, or the natural history of cancer. Treatment experiments for cancers in earlier stages are likely to focus on a cure, whereas MBC clinical trials may be focused on limiting or eliminating further spread of cancer, reducing symptoms, and/or prolonging life.

In this section, we discuss how you can access information about participating in a clinical trial for the treatment and care of MBC. One of the first things you and she should discuss after a diagnosis of MBC is whether to participate in a research clinical trial. Even if she did not explore this option during an earlier stage of her cancer, it is not too late to consider it now. You and she will need some time to absorb the implications of what her oncologist has told her about the spread of the breast cancer to another organ or part of the body, and you will also want the details of the standard treatments being recommended for her at this time. If she is interested in participating in a clinical trial, it is important for her to mention this to her medical team before she starts another treatment for MBC. This is because the inclusion criteria for enrollment in some clinical trials may prioritize patients who can start the experimental trial before any alternative treatment. Yet, even if her treatment is already underway, there may still be research opportunities available to her. Investigating the availability of clinical trials can be a task you can help her with – another form of support, something you can do for her if she would like.

Why would she participate in a clinical trial, especially as no promises are being made it will cure her? There are several reasons. The experimental treatment may turn out to be effective: it could cure the cancer, extend her life by slowing the spread of disease, and/or reduce her symptoms. She could be motivated to participate regardless of personal benefit just to help advance scientific research on cancer causes and cures. Without the voluntary research participation of patients diagnosed with cancer, the medical profession and your local hospital would forever be stuck in the past – using only old treatments from earlier years. New discoveries are only possible through experiments to establish their effectiveness and integrity. Finally, she may want to pursue every avenue available to her, deciding she has nothing to lose and everything to gain. She may even be eager to explore experimental treatments in addition to the treatment options being offered to her by her doctor. Whatever her motivation, you will want to respect her decision.

At any given point in time, there will be dozens of Clinical Trials focused on Metastatic Breast Cancer actively enrolling participants. In the U.S. during February 2021 alone, there were nearly 400 Breast Cancer Clinical Trials, nine of which were new Clinical Trials for Stage IV Breast Cancer that were just starting to recruit volunteer participants. Another 22 trials focused exclusively on MBC began recruitment during the previous two months. You can use search tools on key websites to help narrow down possible options at: https://www.nationalbreastcancer.org/about-breast-cancer/metastatic-trial-search (the National Breast Cancer Foundation, Inc.), and https://www.cancer.gov/about-cancer/treatment/clinical-trials/search (the National Cancer Institute of the National Institutes of Health).

These tools ask for basic information about her cancer, such as the breast cancer biomarkers from her latest biopsy (e.g., ER, PR, HER2, AR); whether the tumor is metaplastic, inflammatory, or lobular; the location in the body where there is evidence of cancer; her birth year; and her zip code to help locate nearby trials. You may already have helped her develop – with her doctor – a treatment summary for ready reference to answer these kinds of questions (See Chapter 2 for a discussion of developing this summary using the ASCO format as a model, pp. 28–32). A copy of a 49-page booklet and forms that can be filed out and edited can be found at https://www.cancer.net/sites/cancer.net/files/cancer_survivorship.pdf. But you can begin the search even if you do not know some of the technical details – "not sure" answers are accepted online. There are also helpful videos you can view before starting your search on both the National Breast Cancer Foundation and the NCI websites:

https://www.cancer.gov/about-cancer/treatment/clinical-trials/search. In addition, the NCI website includes a link for you to connect with someone who will help navigate this process and locate appropriate clinical trials.

Her oncology team can provide more information about clinical trial opportunities – and perhaps even about the specific trials you have identified on the web near you – and answer important questions regarding costs, eligibility criteria, possible benefits, possible risks and side effects, and how these compare with standard treatments available to her locally. Health insurance coverage generally includes costs of a clinical trial, and the research team will have access to grant funds to cover the kinds of costs not covered by health insurance; this could even involve transportation costs where treatments involve regular travel to a research hospital or clinic.

Decisions About Further Treatment

At some point, you and she may be told by her doctors that treatments for her advanced breast cancer are no longer working. They may have shrunk the tumor or slowed its growth, but now even these improvements have stopped. She may still be offered further treatment, but there may be complications. Even with health insurance, the financial costs of more treatment may entail significant sacrifices without enhancing or prolonging her life. Harsh symptoms produced by some treatments can severely compromise her daily life. She may have exhausted opportunities to participate in clinical trial research to try experimental MBC treatments. She may decide to discontinue treatments with side effects that are making her miserable during her remaining time, without any realistic prospect of a cure. Her top priorities may be pain management and leading as normal a life as possible, and she may wish to focus choices on her quality of life and the life of her family, especially children. As we commented in Chapter 3, these are important decisions, made in very stressful times. You can be a caring, educated sounding board to help her think through the costs and benefits of additional treatments. You can support her to make decisions that she feels are best for her.

Quality of Life and Survival During Advanced Cancer

Advancements in the treatment of MBC mean that women are living longer; estimates are that the 5-year survival rate for MBC will double from the current rate of 18% to 36%. Five years or even longer is a long time! Rather than resigning to filling those years with negative thoughts, fears, and the physical and mental consequences of being unwell, there are things you can do to not only help her increase the quantity but also the quality of her life. For example, participation in clinical trial research can give you hope despite the diagnosis.

As we discuss in Chapter 14, there is excellent research on mindfulness showing that learning how to focus on and appreciate what is happening around you now – mindfulness – can reduce symptoms that interfere with daily living such as fatigue, anxiety, depression, sleep disturbances, and even pain. You can help her – and yourself – to step away from distressing thoughts that can creep in, day and night (see Chapter 14, p. 235–236).

She may benefit from the social support of other women with MBC available either face-to-face or online. If the woman you are supporting wants to try participation in such a group, we recommend finding a professionally moderated group rather than a self-help gathering that is not led by a trained facilitator. A professional with experience can mitigate unpleasantness or serious emotional trauma that might emerge under stress during the sharing of negative stories that can cause aversive reactions. Alternatively, she may seek out a Stage IV Breast Cancer Facebook Group (see also Chapter 11) which are more anonymous and can be scheduled at her convenience. A social support group will be beneficial if it helps her to cope. If participation makes her more distressed, she may decide to discontinue this – and that's okay.

Women with MBC often report they look better than they feel so can experience insensitive remarks from others. Because their treatment is ongoing – interspersed with breaks to allow their body some relief from side effects – they may not appear to be suffering from side effects of chemotherapy and radiation such as hair loss, weight loss, fatigue, and nausea. You will know she is not feeling okay and that her many treatments are causing psychological stress, pain, and challenges to managing her health. She may be having trouble sleeping and be depressed. Other family members and friends may not see all of this, so they may think she is fine. What can she say to someone who tells her how great she looks and how lucky she is to be doing so well, when you and she both know how often she feels sick, and her life will never be the same? Hearing remarks like this from someone she knows gives you the opportunity to talk with her about it later. Her preference may be to simply ignore such comments. Or she might appreciate your help in planning how to respond. As this is likely to happen more than once, ask whether there is anything she would like you to do. For example, she might appreciate it if you arrange to speak privately with a friend or family member to explain the situation to them.

Keeping Physically and Mentally Healthy During Treatment for MBC

Physical activity is important for her. Being physically active can help your partner increase her endurance, strengthen muscles and bone, be physically fit, and keep a healthy heart. Muscles, bones, and connective tissues weaken and atrophy when they are not used. She has been ill, so chances are she has not been as physically active as usual. You may still be helping by doing things for her that she used to do on her own, and you may have taken over activities she finds difficult. During her treatment for MBC, you will want to encourage and support her to resume as many normal activities as she can. Falling into a pattern of you now doing all the driving, all the lifting, all the carrying, or not even inviting her to take a walk with you – wanting her to be comfortable in an easy chair – will not be doing her any favors. Help her keep active, as this is something she can control that is extremely important for her overall well-being.

Human movement builds strength and increased range of motion to reach for things and change body position without pain or discomfort. She can build up her strength and stretch her muscles by gradually taking back some of the household chores you, her children, and others might have been doing. Some accommodations will probably be needed: if she cannot bend down to unload the washer and dryer, perhaps she could load the washer and fold the clothes. She could be the one to retrieve the morning paper, benefitting from both the walk and picking it up from the sidewalk or front porch. If you keep doing all the driving – even when she could drive – she will not only become physically uncomfortable but even mentally less able to drive safely. Offer to make a list of the simple everyday chores and activities involving movement, so you and she can keep as fit as possible. Revisit the list regularly, as her situation and tolerance are likely to change over time. This could be a good time to do something together every day to increase her strength and stamina. There are many exercises described on the web that can be done on a yoga mat (they are extremely cheap) or soft carpet on the floor at home – perhaps with a clean beach towel between her and any surface that has come into contact with dirty shoes or sweaty bodies! During the coronavirus pandemic, it was tempting to just sit around and spend days at home reading, watching television, and eating snack foods. Instead, you and she can develop a daily fitness regime that blends easily into daily life.

You and she do not need to launch a formal exercise program by joining a gym or a dance group, but you could take daily walks or do floor exercises when the weather is too awful to go outside. Perhaps you and she had once considered taking dancing lessons: you could check out the options and sign you up for lessons scheduled during her treatment breaks. If you hate dancing but she loves it, you could encourage her to ask a friend to go with her. She could privately share with the teacher that there will be moments when she may need to step away for a few moments to sit and rest. If she has taken some time-off from work during her treatments, she might want to use some of this time doing things she has not had the time to do when she was working full time – gardening, hiking, yoga, swimming, or taking the kids along for long walks with the dog. These are all opportunities for you to help her keep engaged in aspects of her life that are not dominated by cancer.

Encourage her to undertake new hobbies or explore things she used to enjoy. It might be years since she took piano lessons, but playing piano is something she remembers fondly from her childhood. Today's digital pianos and small keyboards (which will be considerably less expensive) come with headphones: practicing will offend no one and give her total freedom to make mistakes without being self-conscious. Bookstores and department stores have a myriad of inexpensive board and card games that could be fun to play with friends and family. An iPad would allow her to spend relaxing time playing Scrabble, Spider, or any of the many free games available online. If you have children or grandchildren, they can show her how to play other electronic games as well. Having a tablet could be good for both of you: Getting up in the middle of the night to spend an hour or so with a boring game of Solitaire on an iPad's nighttime setting can be an excellent way for her to overcome sleeplessness instead of lying wide-awake in bed, worrying.

There are lots of possibilities. She could explore cooking something new once every week or two using a special budget just for that meal. As a teenager, she may have done paint-by-numbers, needlepoint, or used charcoal pencils to draw wintry tree scenes. Ask her if she would like to make a trip with you to the local bookshop, art supply store, or discount store to get her started. Even talking about what might be something new for her to do tomorrow or next week could cheer up both of you!

Palliative and Hospice Care

When advanced breast cancer is no longer responding to treatment and no other treatment options are available, discussing choices for end-of-life care sooner rather than later may make this less painful for her, you, and others in the family. *The most important factor to consider is what is most important to her.* She will need to make decisions about her quality of life, and you must endure the difficult challenge of supporting her decisions even if, in your heart, you disagree. If she wants to live as long as possible, she may want to continue trying aggressive treatments or clinical trials even if they make her uncomfortable and are no longer working. Alternatively, she may want more treatment breaks with a focus on avoiding negative side effects that compromise her time with loved ones. She may prioritize controlling pain and symptoms, and she may tell you she wants to avoid a long process of dying. If you yourself are aware of what is available to her, you can support her decisions about how she prefers to handle this difficult time.

When treatment is no longer an option and not effective, care is available to manage cancer symptoms and make her as comfortable as possible including:

- Palliative Care: Palliative care is designed to help the patient feel better but is not treatment. Some forms of palliative care may begin early, after a diagnosis of advanced cancer, during treatment. Palliative care includes chemotherapy to slow the growth of tumors or surgery to remove those pressing on nerves and causing pain. It may also include professional counseling to deal with emotional issues, spiritual guidance, and help with practical concerns. She may qualify for certain specialized financial assistance to reduce costs to you, including little things such as help with clinic parking fees.
- Hospice Care: Hospice care is provided to patients and their families once further treatment is judged ineffective, life expectancy is 6 months or less, and the emphasis shifts to relieving symptoms and supporting the patient at the end of her life. The major goal is to control pain and

other symptoms to help the person be as comfortable as possible. If the cancer does go into remission, hospice care would stop, and active treatment would resume. Hospice care can happen at home or in a hospital, nursing home, or other specialized facility. Regardless of the location, hospice services may include medical services and supplies; drugs to manage pain and symptoms; physical and occupational therapy; counseling and spiritual advice; social work services; and grief counseling and support. If the patient receives hospice at home, care may also include short-term inpatient care, home health aides, and volunteers to give caregivers a break.

Many countries have government agencies that assist with the cost of such services. In the U.S., Medicare and most Medicaid and health insurance plans cover palliative and hospice care. It will be especially helpful for you to become well informed about the Medicaid and other government benefits available to those who qualify for financial help with medical expenses. This information is typically available from welfare departments in your region, state health departments, state social service agencies, the state Medicaid office, or the health service in other countries. More information about palliative and hospice care is available online at: https://www.cancer.gov/about-cancer/advanced-cancer/care-choices. In the U.S., two other helpful organizations are: National Hospice and Palliative Care Organization http://www.caringinfo.org and the National Association for Home Care & Hospice http://www.nahc.org/.

End-of-Life Planning

For those with MBC, planning for end-of-life care should be in place sooner rather than later. In this section, we describe Advance Directives to protect her wishes and enable her to make her own decisions – to not be cast as a powerless cancer victim with no control over her life. Women with MBC report concerns that their loved ones quite un-derstandably are hesitant to even talk with them about what they want when they are approaching death. Having end-of-life planning in place can help to put her mind at ease. It can reassure her, you, and others in her family that her wishes will be respected.

Reassure your partner she can share her darkest feelings and fears with you at this time. It is impossible to imagine how isolated a woman must feel after being told she is expected to live only a few more months or years. She will need you more than ever, and she will need you to respect whatever decisions she makes for this final stage in her life. You must prepare yourself for what are likely to be very difficult conversations – and for your own sadness as you realize you are losing her.

Luanna's younger sister died at age 45 of breast cancer. MBC can take the lives of women who are even younger than this, women who had every right to imagine a full life ahead. It can take the lives of older women who knew life was not forever but expected to have many more years with their beloved family and friends. Whatever her age, there will be legal and practical issues that you may be able to help her with, and we cover these in the next section.

Financial and Estate Planning

Without going into too much detail here, financial challenges will vary from person to person. The financial burdens and distress accompanying extended treatment for advanced cancer over a period of years has been termed *financial toxicity*, and it is likely to affect all but the wealthiest among us. Cancer patients consistently emphasize the benefits of getting practical financial issues sorted early on. Not putting this off makes it easier to focus on taking care of themselves and their family, without the stress and anxiety of worry about things that do not have to remain unknowns. This section will be most relevant to a spouse or life partner who shares assets and obligations with the patient. If you are a close friend or other family member, you may still be able to help her with some aspects if she seeks your advice. She will be concerned about many issues, so begin – patiently but promptly – to help her plan for the practical issues that you and she can control.

Both you and your partner should already have legal wills on file. If you do not, discuss this with her and help by contacting a lawyer to get this done. Try not to view this as an insensitive reminder of the finality of a diagnosis of MBC, but rather as a way of putting guarantees in place to respect her wishes. You may be confident you have her best interests at heart. But other family members may need the reassurance of legal documentation of agreement about the distribution of her assets (and liabilities). This documentation will be particularly important where minor and/or adult children are involved – including stepchildren if you are a blended family.

In addition to her legal will, encourage her to make a list of the smaller and more personal items she would especially like certain other persons to have – this list should be kept safe along with her legal will. It might include an item of furniture or set of china passed down to her from a grandparent that she wishes a child or grandchild to have. She can decide which precious belongings will be given to all those family members and close friends who will value having something personal to remember her by. Luanna's sister made sure Luanna received the delicate opal necklace that was one of her favorites: for the thirty years since Bonnie's death, this beautiful piece of jewelry has been a treasured reminder of all the good years two sisters enjoyed with one another. You will want to update your lists each year to reflect changes in possessions as well as how you feel about others.

If your home is jointly owned (and possibly mortgaged) by you and her, the death of a spouse can enmesh the survivor legally for months or years waiting for probate to conclude. The best way to protect both of you may be placing ownership of key assets – such as your house – into a trust. Revocable or irrevocable trusts, written individually for you and your wife, are relatively commonplace and easily arranged with legal advice. Joint savings and checking accounts, credit cards, retirement accounts, and other shared assets can suddenly become complicated for you to access. You can also help your partner by organizing records, insurance policies, documents, and instructions and keeping original copies of important documents in a fireproof box or safe as well as with a lawyer when appropriate, including key passwords. Pull out materials you think might be relevant and important and go through materials with her. Offer to take responsibility for distributing needed copies to family members. These can include birth and marriage certificates, adoption papers, and any genetic and/or genealogical information she has stored. If you have a safe deposit box for valuables and important documents, make sure someone else in the family besides you – with her consent – has access. This may also be the time she chooses to discard communications or records from the past that may involve private and personal matters she now wants kept in the past, not passed on to family after her death.

Planning for Children and the Family

There is something particularly tragic and sad about a mom with young children facing the reality of MBC. If you are the father or mother of those children, you will be facing the reality of one day raising them without her. This inevitable emotional turmoil for you and your children cannot be willed away or swept under the rug. The final section of this chapter will address strategies you and she might find helpful to manage your emotions and reactions during these final years, months, weeks, and days (see also Chapter 14). But sharing a home and children with your spouse or partner means you must plan – with her – for what will happen after she is gone.

There is research showing that after a diagnosis of MBC, mothers worry most about the care of their children after their death. Research studies also have found that moms report knowing their young children will be well cared for after they die is more calming and reassuring than anything else. If you and the woman you love are the parents of children still living at home, her diagnosis could lead you to make some lifestyle changes to help to put her mind at ease about their future. For example – and this could be just a relevant for an early-stage cancer diagnosis – you could decide to play a larger role in the children's lives beyond the kinds of activities you typically share with them. If your children view her as the major nurturing parent in your home, can you step up emotionally to share this role? She needs your reassurance that you will be committed to the children and their future no matter what, that you will make sure they feel loved and cared for all their lives. There may also be big decisions you have discussed but not done anything about, such as making a move to a more manageable home or even to a different geographical location closer to grandparents and other family members. While a move can be disruptive for you and your children – involving them changing schools and leaving friends – there may be accommodations you can make such as coordinating a move with transitions across different levels of schooling. If this is something you have talked about even before her cancer diagnosis, now could be the right time to plan and take the necessary steps.

Facing issues such as these – letting her know and showing her that you will do your best – could make a huge difference to her peace of mind.

Advance Directives

One of your first steps in end–of–life planning should be ensuring you and she have your Advance Medical Directives, Advance Health Care Directives, or Living Wills in place. These are different terms for legal documents giving directions to health care providers and others involved in caring for a terminally ill person. An Advance Directive template will be available from her health care provider to complete for specific choices in medical emergencies. Once you and your wife know that her death is not just possible but probable, making these decisions while she can think clearly about what is most important gives her more control over this end stage in her life. Ideally, you should both prepare legally binding Advance Directives long before being diagnosed with a terminal illness. But if your partner has not done so, this should be one of the first things you both do following a diagnosis of MBC.

If you are her husband, wife, or partner, we recommend you do this together – one for each of you, not just for her – long before her medical team has told her that treatments are no longer working, and that she may have only a few more months to live. It can be stressful for both of you to make decisions about final orders for life-saving medical treatment right after being told there are no longer any options available to treat her cancer. You can help by not only getting the information and template form for her, but by completing a document for yourself as well.

If you and she have waited until the last minute, it will be tempting to avoid this process and continue waiting. Waiting too long can have serious consequences because medical doctors are sworn to do whatever they can to save a life – even if death is inevitable. Without an Advance Directive with specific instructions, emergency and hospital staff are required to intervene during a medical emergency and do whatever they can to keep her alive. Life-saving emergency measures can seriously and permanently compromise any remaining quality time she could otherwise spend with family, and she should have the choice to decide what she wants or does not want done in such an emergency. Cardiopulmonary resuscitation (CPR) can result in a broken sternum or ribs; intubation on a ventilator requires sedation and physical restraint; and insertion of a feeding tube as substitute for taking food by mouth can sustain life long after brain activity has ceased.

An Advance Directive with alternative instructions can be revised or revoked at any time. A properly constituted Advance Directive will direct health care providers and others to provide, withhold, or withdraw treatment in accordance with specified choices. The document is likely to begin with the choice of either prolonging life whenever possible or not to prolong life if the person has an incurable condition that will result in death within a short period of time, has become unconscious in what is judged by medical personnel as a permanent state, or when the likely risks and effects of treatment outweigh the expected benefits.

A second proviso will enable the signer to choose whether nutrition and/or hydration should be provided, regardless of whether she has chosen to prolong life or not intervene medically to do so. A third choice will involve relief from pain, choosing whether to receive or decline pain relief if it hastens death. The Advance Directive will also document someone as her health care power of attorney who can make decisions on her behalf as an agent who vows to consider her personal values. You may be her primary agent in most cases, and there may be an adult daughter or son she would name as her second (alternate) agent should you be unable to do this at the time.

Once this legal document is completed, ensure that health care providers have a copy on file. She (both of you if you are married or partners) should also keep a copy in a secure but accessible location at home, as there could come a time when emergency medical personnel arrive and would otherwise begin the exact procedures that are not wanted. In that case, you will need to show them her Advance Directive on the spot. Also, it is important to give a copy to any other family member who needs to have it. This should minimally include adult children most likely to survive you and your wife. If they have a copy, they will know what their mother wants even if she is no longer able to tell them. Her wishes can only be respected if others know what they are!

Death with Dignity

At the time we were writing this book, eight states and the District of Columbia have passed a Death with Dignity Act. This allows a terminally ill person to end their life through voluntary self-administration of a lethal dose of medication prescribed by a doctor. Originally passed as a citizens' initiative in the 1994 general election and later reaffirmed by referendum in 1997, the Oregon Death with Dignity Act (DWDA) is a model for similar legislation in other locales. It has been in place long enough to provide reassurance of protections against abuses including medical malfeasance or unfair pressures on a vulnerable patient by family members. There may come a time when she wants to explore this option and take charge of her death rather than succumbing slowly (and even painfully) to the timetable of the cancer. If she is considering medical assistance in dying, you may be called upon to show exceptional courage in supporting her decision – and perhaps even being at her side when the time comes.

Medical aid in dying for those who are terminally ill is legal under well-specified circumstances in many countries. In addition to nearly a dozen states in the US, other nations that have passed similar legislation include Canada, Belgium, the Netherlands, Luxembourg, Switzerland, Germany, Australia, New Zealand, and Portugal. The Death with Dignity National Center in the US hosts a website that tracks the status of these laws, so you can find out what exists in your state: https://www.deathwithdignity.org/take-action.

Her Legacy

Throughout our lives, most of us do not probe deeply into the meaning of life. That may be wise given limitations on what we know, what we can do, and what is even possible. When someone is approaching the end of their own life, however, they can take charge of something we all care about: our legacy.

Someone who knows they are dying will want closure for some things and to open doors for others. Those who have never been close to death cannot really know what this is like, but human beings value the final stage of life as a time for being at peace with the world and with oneself. They may seek to mend old fences; renew friendships from the past; do things they never dared previously to do; seek forgiveness from family and their God for things they regret; and – especially – enjoy as much quality time as they have remaining with those they love. Those who die unexpectedly do not have these opportunities, but someone who is terminally ill does.

If you're her husband, wife, or partner, there will be practical issues you and she may have settled long ago, such as whether you wished to be buried or cremated after death. You may have discussed (and even perhaps put this in a legal document so your children know) where you want to be buried or your ashes to be scattered. You and she may have signed agreements to donate your bodies to a medical school. Ideally, these will not be issues you have to talk about now – all the more reason why we should all do advance planning for the inevitable long before we are close to the end of our lives.

Finally, the remaining weeks, months, or even years of her life should be about creating her legacy. How can you support her to make her legacy, to tell the story of her life the way she wishes to be remembered? When hope for life can otherwise be slipping away, she can hope to leave behind a legacy to acknowledge a life well lived. Some of the things that may give her pleasure to prepare and solace to others later, after she is gone, include:

* *Her story*: She can write her own story for you to keep and to share with others. This may even be the basis of her obituary. Otherwise, her obituary will be written by well-meaning family members who can name surviving family members but may not know much about accomplishments she is proud of. She can also select the photo she wishes her local newspaper to use.
* *Planning her service*: She may want a traditional funeral, or she may prefer what is called a Celebration of Life. When it feels safe to talk about this, ask her what she wants to do and what this should be like, what music should be played, and whom to invite. You might have this conversation when hospice care begins, and you should talk about it on more than one occasion so she can think about what

she wants. Keep notes and then, when she has decided on important details, print out what you understand her wishes to be and show this to her so she can be certain.

- *Letters to those who are special to her:* She could compose letters to you, her children, her parents, and any others special to her that she would like them to read in the future. For example, it can be sad but also uplifting to be able to give a son or daughter a sealed envelope containing a special note on their wedding day or upon the birth of their first child: *Mom is not here, but if I were, this is what I would want to tell you.* There may even be a letter for you, and you will have to resist any temptation to open and read it until the time she specified.

- *Reading:* There may be books she always wanted to read but never had time to finish. She may also want to re-read books she read as a child or young adult. You can help by ordering these for her in a format she can handle, in print or on Kindle.

- *Writing, favorite quotes, and thoughts:* She may enjoy having a personal notebook, diary, or recorder to save thoughts that come to her, quotes that impress her, and even a poem or two. Poetry does not have to meet anyone else's standards but our own to be meaningful! She could record what is called an "ethical will" of her values, hopes, and dreams, to pass on to others.

- *Making playlists of favorite songs:* There are electronic devices you can use to help her make a playlist of her favorite songs or even multiple playlists for different moods. These could be playlists she will enjoy now but later pass on to someone else – you, a child, or a close friend whom she has known for years.

- *Sorting through mementos and old photos:* There are few things as tiring, dusty, and taxing as going through boxes of unsorted family materials to try to put them in order. You and anyone else who is willing can be a big help by getting things started: you can separate different types of things, sort photos by categories that make sense (e.g., her own childhood versus each of her own children's photos), and clean out any silverfish that have crept into the corners! You could set up a manageable number of items for her to sort through in a place that will be comfortable for her, have some idea of how long she can do this before becoming tired, then reappear when she needs a break to help put everything away.

- *Gathering favorite recipes:* Together, you could make a list of favorite foods and meals across the years, and together you can recall where to find the recipe. You could enlist help from her family, adult children, or a close friend – as all you may have to do is hand them a pile of cookbooks and list of recipes. They can do the work! The result could be an electronic recipe 'cookbook' to share with family and friends.

- *Making a family tree*: In the days of DNA testing through Ancestry.com and 23AndMe there are multiple options to learn about one's ethnic make-up, something that could be of interest to her and her children. The test kits require only a bit of saliva, and the resulting report can be fascinating. This could also lead to creating a Family Tree with help from someone in the family who agrees to keep this archive.

- *Writing her autobiography*: Not everyone is a writer or enjoys writing, but those memories and photographs could form the core of her autobiography. Looking back, we have all lost family members and realized how little we really knew about their lives. Luanna's father spent several years writing his own autobiography: before he died, she had it printed and bound – photographs included – for him to enjoy and to share with the rest of the family. His memories may not always have been accurate, but they describe a life well lived, and even Luanna's adult daughter loved having a copy.

- *Making special gifts to loved ones*: We mentioned this earlier, but she will have little things that are special to her that she will want passed on to someone in the family or a close friend. You could make sure you know what these are and either keep a list for later reference, or, if she prefers, organize the times and places for her to pass these things along now, herself.

These are only a few ideas for how you can support your wife, partner, loved one, or the person you care about to create a legacy – to tell her story to others in as many ways as she chooses. She will know which make sense to her. Above all else, this will be about her and the legacy she wishes to leave behind.

Summary and Recommendations

- Be prepared for the possibility that your wife, partner, loved one, or the person you care about could develop MBC as long as ten years after an early-stage breast cancer was treated. While MBC is a worst-case scenario, becoming informed can mean many more years of a good quality of life, and you can help her plan for this.
- Know the symptoms of MBC and encourage her to share signs with you and go to her doctor with concerns.
- If she has not done this already, encourage her (and her husband or wife if this is not you) to prepare wills and advance directives, sort

financial matters, and ask her doctor to complete a cancer summary and treatment history. Make copies of relevant documents available to key family members.

- You can help her locate opportunities to participate in clinical trial research exploring new treatments for MBC and discuss these with her oncology team.
- Every so often, talk with her about how she is feeling and whether she is managing her symptoms. Encourage her to seek additional advice from her doctor if you notice increases in her pain and discomfort.
- If she chooses to participate in a support group for women with MBC, support her decision and suppress any temptation to feel you need to know everything about what she is saying and doing.
- Explore different ways you can both remain active and physically healthy despite her cancer. Her cancer, treatment, and symptoms may limit what she can do, but with your support she can resume many activities to be as physically fit as possible.
- Be mindful and help her to be mindful of the beautiful moments and special people all around her.
- Support her to look for new opportunities to engage in activities that interest her, perhaps things she always wanted but never had time to do. This includes hobbies and activities to do with you, by herself, and with others.
- Be brave in helping her to weigh the relative costs and benefits of each treatment decision, for her personally and for the future of her children, other family members, and you.
- Help her create a personally meaningful legacy to share for many years to come, one that celebrates her life and love.

Sources for More Information

Awan, A. A., Hutton, B., Hilton, J., Mazzarello, S., Van Poznak, C., & Vandermeer, L. (2019). De-escalation of bone-modifying agents in patients with bone metastases from breast cancer: a systematic review and meta-analysis. *Breast Cancer Research and Treatment, 176*, 507–517. https://dx.doi.org.helicon.vuw.ac.nz/10.1 007/s10549-019-05265-1

Barney, A. (2020). *When life hands you cactuses, make margaritas.* Life Lessons Publishing.

Kashian, N., & Jacobson, S. (2020). Factors of engagement and patient-reported outcomes in a Stage IV breast cancer Facebook group. *Health Communication, 35*, 75–82. 10.1080/10410236.2018.1536962.

Lundquist, D. M., Berry, D. L., Boltz, M., DeSanto-Madeya, S. A., & Grace, P. J. (2019). Wearing the mask of wellness: The experience of young women living with advanced breast cancer. *Oncology Nursing Forum, 46*, 329–337. 10.1188/1 9.onf.329-337.

Jung, M. Y., & Matthews, A. K. (2021). A systematic review of clinical interventions facilitating end-of-life communication between patients and family caregivers. *American Journal of Hospice & Palliative Medicine, 38*:2, 180–190.

Yee, J., Davis, G. M., Beith, J. M., Wilcken, N., Currow, D., Emery, J. ... Kilbreath, S. L. (2014). Physical activity and fitness in women with metastatic breast cancer. *Journal of Cancer Survivorship, 8*, 647–656.

Zimmaro, L. A., Carson, J. W., Olsen, M. K., Sanders, L., Keefe, F. J., & Porter, L. S. (2020). Greater mindfulness associated with lower pain, fatigue, and psychological distress in women with metastatic breast cancer. *Psycho-Oncology, 29*, 263–270. https://doi-org.helicon.vuw.ac.nz/a0.1002/pon.5223

14 Taking Care of You

Thus far in this book everything is about what you can do for the person you are caring for, as well as your children and family if you are her partner, so you can be fully informed about breast cancer and work collaboratively with medical professionals. That seems like you're expected to be Superman or Wonder Woman! But as you're probably not a superhero, this chapter is strictly about what you can do for yourself. This is not selfish. The quality of support and care you can offer her is dependent on you staying strong, healthy, and capable. If you fall apart, you can't be much help to anyone else. And it's a well-known fact that your stress level affects the stress level of the person you are caring for.

Much of the research we draw on for this chapter is based on conversations and reports from both male and female intimate partners of women with breast cancer. For convenience, we will sometimes refer to you as her partner (spouse, husband, or wife). But we fully recognize you might be a friend or a close relative. Some of the examples we offer and situations we describe, therefore, might be a little different from your specific circumstances, but the principles of self-care will be similar.

You might be surprised to learn there has been a great deal of research carried out on people exactly like you – someone taking on the role of primary caregiver. And the picture emerging is not an entirely happy one. Some people say the overall experience of caring for a person with cancer had beneficial elements for them (we'll mention these later). But the majority of research participants say they experienced anxiety and worry, depression, economic challenges, reduced quality of life, guilt, frustration, paranoia, and, in the case of married couples, dissatisfaction with the relationship and interference with sexuality. The more distressed you are, the more likely you are to overestimate her level of distress, anxiety, and depression. She may prefer practical help, not just emotional support. Care-giving partners tended to underestimate their own needs. These needs were for information, dealing with sexuality,

DOI: 10.4324/9781003194088-14

daily living needs, and technical knowledge about how to provide physical care. Men especially tend to overstate their level of adjustment and coping ability, but whatever your gender don't think you're tough and can do it all!

In this chapter, therefore, we offer practical suggestions for how to keep mentally and physically healthy, how to cope with challenging situations and feelings, and how to manage your own stress levels for the good of you, her, and everyone else in the family. Neither we nor you can wave a magic wand and expect life to be hunky dory from now on. Just think how much has been written in a large array of self-help books about "how to stop worrying and start living," "overcoming depression," "don't sweat the small stuff," "fighting anxiety," "the art of mindfulness," "change your brain," "finding emotional resilience," "running for mental health" – the titles are endless. Self-help books can be useful, but we're not preaching, selling one approach, or telling you exactly what to do. We offer some simple suggestions and reminders which others in your situation – including ourselves – have found useful.

If You've Had Bad Days, You're Not Alone

Let's start the discussion with the known risks to your well-being when you become a major support for a woman with breast cancer. If you have or are likely to experience any of these reactions, you can be sure you're not the first.

The most general thing to recognize is that from the moment you hear she's been diagnosed with breast cancer you are under a new disruptive form of stress, both physical and mental. Humans' response to stress is well understood – there are physiological changes interfering with every aspect of your bodily functions. These reactions might include increased blood pressure (hypertension); migraines; muscle tension headaches; sleep problems; aches and pains such as joint pain and back pain; non-cardiac chest pain; heart palpitations; loss of appetite and indigestion; irregular bowel movements or diarrhea. These stress reactions can then cause further difficulties, such as eating problems (overeating or not eating balanced meals), fatigue, feeling on edge, and being moody and erratic in your behavior. In research studies, some spouses of women with breast cancer have reported excessive worry about their own health and even imagine symptoms of cancer in themselves.

At the same time, your thoughts can also be in turmoil. You might be worrying about your partner, or having to take time off work, or how to support her, what to say and not say to her and others, and how much her treatment will cost. These are the sorts of things we often ruminate about, especially when trying to fall asleep. Running all these worries through your head makes it harder to sleep. Then, if you become less rested and more fatigued, you have a new worry – about not sleeping or having disturbing dreams and nightmares. Attempting to stay cheerful and positive for her sake might make you less likely to talk with her about your feelings, which you try to bottle up. Feeling guilty about your own good health when she is so sick might not make you more understanding of what your partner is going through, but less so. That in turn can make you impatient or quick to take offence.

It is also possible areas of conflict you have had in your relationship with her will be more evident, no matter how hard you try to overlook them. When you are under stress, it is not uncommon to talk to someone in ways that reveal some degree of underlying resentment or irritation. This is a phenomenon called "expressed [negative] emotion." A good example might be making a nasty remark supposedly as a joke.

In summary, the most common mental health problems reported by partners of women with breast cancer are anxiety, depression, irritability, fear of loss, doubts about the relationship, and difficulty thinking flexibly in a way that can solve problems. Negative feelings are very un- comfortable. None of us like them, so we all are susceptible to conscious and unconscious efforts to keep them away.

Things we do to manage our negative feelings include actions like drinking more alcohol, smoking more than usual, binge eating snack food, trying to deny your feelings, and avoiding situations and con- versations that might set them off. In Chapter 1 we described such efforts as coping attempts that are potentially dysfunctional – they make matters worse. In Chapter 12 on supporting your children, we summarized more positive ways of coping with stress and negative feelings. If you don't have children in the family you might have skipped that chapter, so it might be a good idea to go back and read the couple of pages on coping strategies (pp. 186–188) – they apply to grownups just as much as they do to children. Attempting to focus on your emotions or deny them as a way of coping can offer a short-term remedy. But they're not likely to be permanent solutions, especially as they then create other problems further on.

You Have to Take Care of Yourself

Doing what you can for your own mental health and quality of life is being sensible, not self-centered. You've probably heard the standard command from flight attendants when explaining the safety features of the plane just before take-off: "Please put on your own oxygen mask before helping others such as your children." Obviously if you're gasping for air, you can't help the passenger next to you. The same principle applies to you and the person you are supporting. If you are a psychological mess and are falling apart, what degree of real support can you offer her? Research has shown that the greater a caregiver's burden, the more distress, anxiety, depression, and family problems were reported by the individual being supported by that caregiver. Everyone in a family or friendship network is psychologically inter-connected.

So here are some simple starting rules for self-care:

- *Don't be a martyr.* This means don't immediately give up all sorts of things you usually enjoy. You'll have to make lots of accommodations for her, but make sure you leave time for your own activities. A simple rule is to ensure you do at least one thing for yourself every week, which could be something you like to do by yourself.
- *Maintain your own social connections and friendships.* This means you should do things with friends that you have done in the past – meet in a bar, attend your coffee klatch, play poker, have a round of golf, get a pedicure, go bowling after work, stick with your Saturday morning running group, keep up your Facebook friends.... You get the idea. Find a way to continue doing the social activities you typically enjoy, whatever they are. If you usually go to church or temple on a regular basis, keep doing so. Don't apologize to your partner for leaving for a few hours (when the time to do so is okay). Chatting to your friends, expressing your worries, talking to your parents or adult children on the phone or by video chat (like FaceTime), are all opportunities for venting, sorting out muddled ideas, or getting reassuring feedback and encouragement from others. It's the coping strategy we call social support.
- *Keep physically fit.* Go to the gym; don't give it up. Go for brisk walks by yourself. Take the kids for a bike ride. Unless your work already requires a great deal of movement, do one physical activity every day. Lots of research supports the physical, psychological, and emotional benefits of regular exercise, so we'll say more about this later.
- *An apple a day ... et cetera.* Be sure to eat healthy foods – you know the things that are bad for you! Take a multivitamin, even if you think you don't need one.
- *New activities.* If you've had to take time off work temporarily, you'll find yourself with an unusual amount of down-time at home. You're likely to be spending hours waiting in clinic and hospital settings for her cancer appointments and treatments – you could take along an electronic tablet to play Solitaire to help pass the time.

It's not uncommon to feel you don't have any time for yourself now you're so busy with all the extra chores and duties and child-care. These things are all about good time management and creating new windows of opportunity: find a new hobby, read books or e-books, listen to music with earbuds or headphones so others aren't bothered, play card games or board games with the kids or others, go for scenic drives, or suggest other quiet activities you can do with her.

• *Self-reinforcement (rewarding yourself)*. In Chapter 12, we encouraged you to use lots of rewards – "reinforcements" – for your children's good behavior. The same principle applies to you. But self-reinforcement needs to be more structured; you need to specify in advance what actions deserve a reward and what that reward should be. After doing some task – maybe not your most preferred activity – give yourself a tangible reward. You could buy something just for you; rent a good movie on television; get tickets for a football game you'd love to attend but can't usually afford to. Make a list of your favorite things and prepare to splurge on yourself after you have done something well, hard, or disliked. No cheating! This only works if your self-reinforcement is truly deserved.

Drilling a Little Deeper

All of the above strategies are rather basic and easily done. You should give yourself permission to do things that you enjoy so you can stay healthy. But every problem won't be solved with basic self-care. In the next section, we discuss how to deal constructively with thoughts and emotions that cannot be simply pushed away.

Guilt

It may seem odd to feel guilty over something that is absolutely not your fault. But survivor guilt is a common phenomenon in people who have survived a traumatic experience when others have not. Possibly you've heard of it in connection with combat veterans who have witnessed the death of fellow soldiers. The thought is "Why them, not me?" and that's exactly what some people experience thinking of the serious illness of someone they care deeply about. You may feel you don't deserve to be so healthy.

The problem with survivor guilt is that unlike feeling guilty for something you did wrong, you can't escape it by making amends. There are, however, some things you can do if you are experiencing survivor guilt. Remind yourself that no one is to blame – cancer isn't a punishment for bad behavior. Think about your own health as a gift. Yes, your partner has had bad luck, but bad luck is purely random. There is a well-known book called "When Bad Things Happen to Good People" written by Harold Kushner, a rabbi. If you are a religious or spiritual person you too might question why God let something terrible happen to her when she is such a wonderful person. It is easier for those with strong faith to think that things happen for a reason, and that God has a purpose – an example of a coping strategy we called "meaning-making coping" in Chapter 12. Also, if you believe God regulates our lives, you might start to believe your partner *has* done something wrong and is being punished for it. What Rabbi Kushner suggested is that you can still believe in God's power but realize that the laws of nature and human evolution complicate things. Rabbi Kushner's main message was not to question your faith, but to accept what has happened and decide what constructive actions you can take now and in the future.

If you tend to look for scientific explanations then you may believe the universe has no inherent purpose or design – much of what happens to us is random and uncontrollable. This results in the same conclusion regarding taking action: do something you can control, don't fret over what you can't. Think, for instance, of the kindness and care the medical staff is offering your partner and make it a goal to act with reciprocal kindness and humanity.

Anxiety

Anxiety is different from fear, which is the intense emotional reaction that occurs when you are facing a real danger. The physiological changes that constitute fear (increased heartbeat, rapid breathing, sweaty palms, tensed muscles, nausea, and a sudden urge to defecate or urinate) were all designed in evolution for us to respond to the danger – to be instantly prepared to either fight or flee. Anxiety, on the other hand, occurs when there is a *threat* of possible danger or harm in the future, or you expect something bad. As you don't know when or where the danger might be coming from, fearful bodily reactions aren't much use – you don't need them at that moment, but your body responds as if you do. These distant threats might be related to harmful things that could happen to your partner rather than you. They can also be part of impending crises, such as financial difficulties. This kind of anxiety is similar to worrying about something that is improbable but not impossible. Mistakenly judging the likelihood of improbable or implausible events can be a major cause of anxiety.

The feelings of anxiety and worry are unpleasant and do not help you to confront a realistic danger by running away (flight) or counter-attacking (fight). These unpleasant feelings typically motivate (lead to) actions to reduce them – doing something to avoid the anxious feelings. Avoidance behavior includes things like taking the stairs instead of using the elevator if you dread getting trapped in one, not going on a vacation if you are anxious about flying, or getting someone else to do your shopping if you are nervous in crowded places. Avoidance might also include dodging anxious thoughts by not putting them into words or putting off tasks that make you nervous, like going to the dentist.

The trouble is, of course, by avoiding and not confronting anxiety-provoking situations, you never give anxiety a chance to fade away, or for you to discover your worries were illogical, or unnecessary, or that your negative predictions of what might happen were simply wrong. In the last section of this chapter, we discuss the importance of neither avoiding anxious feelings nor fighting them all the time. Just accept them for what they are – thoughts, not reality – and do your best not to actively avoid situations that might cause you anxiety. Don't shy away from intense experiences that are part of living, whether good or bad. Remember the old principle that if you fall off a bicycle you have to get back on, not give up riding!

But anxiety can also be what we call free-floating, just a general vague sense of dread. The trigger for this is usually uncertainty – not knowing what might happen next, whether she will get sicker or die – or feeling a total lack of control over all possible outcomes. Both those conditions are pretty typical of life when supporting someone with breast cancer, are they not? So, uncertainty and lack of control are potentially harmful to your overall feelings of wellbeing.

Research has shown that people's personalities differ in terms of their ability to live with uncertainty – good for you if you can do so. For most of us, however, the best antidote to chronic insecurity and doubts is to create reliable routines and events that are under our control and thus predictable. At the same time, have back-up plans if a possibly unforeseen event does occur. Let us offer one example – it might not be that relevant to you, but it will give you an idea of the strategy. Let's say you live far from the nearest town hospital, in a cold climate where it often snows. There will be times when she might need to go suddenly to the hospital emergency room. Be prepared: simple basic things like keep your gas tank reasonably full, put on snow tires each winter, carry kitty litter and a snow-shovel in your trunk, keep your driveway clear. But also put in place Plan B: talk to your neighbor who has a 4 × 4 truck and explain your anxiety. In an emergency, would he or she be willing in the middle of the night to help you out with a ride into town? Some partners have reported a form of anxiety that could be called suspiciousness. It is easy to get a bit paranoid when you're worried about your partner. "Are the doctors really doing their best?" "Are there better treatments at other hospitals?" "Surely this medicine can't cost that much – are the drug companies trying to rip me off?" We have often encouraged you, throughout this book, to ask questions like this (but *not* in these exact and hostile words!). One of the things you will come to appreciate with all your new involvements with critical health care is the incredible, unselfish dedication of medical staff. But if you *are* worried and can't shake off the feeling, ask your questions in a respectful way – you will discover the training, ethics, and scientific integrity of doctors and nurses is truly extraordinary.

Depression

Depression is a state of being which can range from being down in the dumps or in a bad mood, to much more serious and chronic feelings of despair, hopelessness, and unworthiness. The condition of "clinical depression" is at the most negative end of that scale. Our suggestions in this section are known to be helpful at all levels of depression. But if you find you cannot shake off the feelings or the things you have tried to improve your mood have not worked, then you should seek professional advice. Struggling with serious depression on your own can impair your own functioning and quality of life and make it difficult for you to provide care to the person you are supporting.

One of the best known and most extensively researched theories of depression has been developed by the psychiatrist Aaron T. Beck. Many scholarly books have been written about his ideas, but the essence of his theory is quite simple. Basically, he argued the feeling of depression is not triggered by objectively terrible things happening to you. If you feel sad because of the loss of a friend or a pet or a failure at work, then you have a perfectly good reason to be sad, to grieve, and to be unhappy. That is not a mental health problem. But if you are depressed because things don't *seem* to be going right for you, those depressed feelings arose because of the thoughts you had and the things you've been saying to yourself. Beck called these "automatic thoughts" – and some people seem to be prone to engage in these negative thoughts more readily than others.

The key thing to understand is that these negative thoughts are not based on reality. If you have one bad experience or failure and you say to yourself, "I'm worthless," that is obviously not true. If you are criticized by a friend and you think, "Everyone hates me," that too is obviously untrue. And if you face some sort of difficulty or barrier in your life and you say to yourself, "It's hopeless, things will never get better," that is rarely true in life. If you say, "Everything in this town sucks, the climate's getting worse, the neighborhood is full of crime," that appraisal is too general despite some elements of truth. Dr. Beck suggested there are three domains or issues people can feel depressed about: themselves, the future, and the world they live in. In the list of common irrational or very biased thoughts we've just given, you will see examples from all three of these domains.

Mental health professionals who follow an effective therapeutic approach called cognitive behavior therapy (CBT) have techniques for changing these irrational thoughts. You can't just say to someone "Stop thinking in that negative way!" Mostly these techniques involve careful persuasive reasoning, helping people see that their thoughts are not based on reality. Depressed individuals are asked to practice at home by consciously repeating more positive things to themselves. Sometimes they will be given little exercises to check on the reality of their negative expectations. Sometimes a client will be asked to write a letter to themselves in which only realistic positive ideas are expressed; the letter might include a list of negative thoughts followed by more accurate alternatives. A professional therapist will also recommend "behavioral activation" – don't sit around in the dark moping; get up and out and do something. Seriously depressed people will say they have no energy or get no pleasure from activities they once enjoyed. The therapist will ask them to start off doing some small thing. If it goes well, then gradually get back to doing and getting pleasure from previous activities.

You can do some of these same things yourself. If one of your children asks you to do something with them when you're in a depressed mood, you might refuse. Catch yourself saying "no," "can't," "maybe next week," and immediately suggest an alternative instead – the simplest thing you're willing to do. If that goes well, agree to a bigger activity the next time. You can also check on whether your most negative thoughts are based on reality by reading reliable, research-based material such as we cover in this book, rather than focusing on wild ideas floating around on social media. You can practice saying more positive words to yourself, by keeping a diary and writing down each evening one really positive event, thought, or experience that happened that day – and then share it with the person you are caring for. If you expect the people on her medical team to ignore you or be upset with your questions, try an experiment: ask them directly if they are comfortable with all your queries and issues you raise.

Avoidance

Your anxiety and depression associated with her breast cancer can result in your avoidance of awkward, painful, or distressing conversations and activities that could potentially help her cope with her diagnosis and treatment. You can see how a tendency on your part to avoid unpleasantness can lead you to disengage from her and her illness at the very time that involvement and action are needed most.

Breast cancer, unlike other chronic illnesses such as diabetes or multiple sclerosis, can evoke mental images of painful death and disfigurement. Some try to conceal their fears she might die and their sadness and horror for what might lie ahead. This kind of avoidance and stoicism takes emotional and mental effort, which prevents the couple from understanding each other fully. Sometimes having a good cry, either alone or with her, is a helpful way to relieve tension.

Anger and Irritability

One of the things we know is that stressful situations, such as caring for someone with a serious illness, can cause or increase feelings of anger and irritability. Men seem particularly susceptible to exploding with anger in response to threat. Remember our mention of "fight or flight" when facing threat — anger is an emotion underlying wanting to fight. We all know that. We also learn throughout our lives to resist aggression by controlling and managing our anger. We learn to take a deep breath, to walk away from a provocative situation, to react assertively but not violently, and to talk to oneself ("relax; stay calm; don't let this get to you; take your inner kettle off the boil; you can work this out a better way").

The stress of caring for her, with all the associated worry and disruptions to your life, is unlikely to trigger physical aggression. But you could get angry in frustrating situations, lose your temper, bang things around, shout at the kids, and get upset with other perfectly innocent people. If that happens, it is helpful to remember these are common human reactions to feeling you are in a threatening or highly aversive situation you cannot control. Use the simple anger management techniques mentioned above and apologize to the children or other persons to whom your anger was directed: "I'm so sorry. I just lost it for a moment. Things have been tough, but I'm not blaming anyone. I'm going to do better." Whatever words come naturally to you and the situation.

Angry outbursts in which you feel rage or fury and want to strike out are usually short, intense, and out of proportion to the actual threat or blocking of your goals and intentions. Irritability is in some ways a minor form of anger, but it is more akin to feeling disgruntled or annoyed when everything seems to be going wrong. Irritability is not usually directed at any one cause; it colors everything you are experiencing. When you recognize what is going on inside you resulting in a grumpy mood, remind yourself it is the unfair, regrettable, unpleasant things happening around that are making you feel this way.

Some people are more susceptible to responding with irritation to frustrating, stressful circumstances. But for her sake, you should try to catch yourself in such a mood, accept that it is natural in such a circumstance and deliberately get yourself out if it. You could use humor – you can't feel irritable and be laughing at the same time, especially when laughing at oneself. Look for the funny side of a situation and talk about it. Tell a joke; hum a song. Smile more often. Think to yourself of all the blessings in your life. Stop what you're doing and do something else. Be mindful – savor the world around you. Hug her and your other loved ones. Give everyone ice cream. Some of these suggestions are much better than others, but they all rely on doing something positive as an alternative to bad feelings.

Positive Alternatives

Rather than dwelling on all the problems and difficulties confronting you, we want to emphasize the positive things you can do to stay strong. In this section we are going to describe some of the beneficial steps you can take – sort of "Eat your vegetables!" advice for the mind.

Among the easiest to establish as a routine (see Chapter 12 for a discussion of routines) is regular exercise. That doesn't necessarily mean sweating it out on a treadmill in a gym – although if you can access a gym and enjoy serious workouts we're happy to encourage you to continue. But even a simple daily walk or bicycle ride or swim at your local rec center is tremendously valuable for both body and mind. And if you prefer to be less public and more socially distanced, there are many good YouTube programs for you to do on the floor at home.

Being able to clear your mind of stressful, sad, and worrying thoughts is clearly the best antidote to persistent negative feelings and the best way to allow your body to quit being constantly prepared only for "fight or flight." Being physically relaxed and calm is the opposite – the positive alternative – of being tense and upset, and fortunately you can deliberately do things which relax you and reduce tension. There are hundreds of different possible ways for you to do this. We tend to think the ones you usually do when on vacation or when you get home from work or when you go out for a good time with friends or family are the ones you should continue to do. This might be sitting in the sun with a cold drink, lying on the sand at a beach, plonked out in your recliner chair with a good movie on TV and a big bowl of popcorn with a lot of melted butter, sitting in the lotus position and repeating your mantra, or going to a licensed massage therapist. Whatever works for you have to find a little time each week to do it. Somewhat more concretely, we are going to comment on sleep, relaxation, meditation, acceptance, and mindfulness. It's all about clearing your head and staying healthy.

Sleep

A tendency to ruminate is one of the better known challenges for people heavily involved in loving care for someone with breast cancer. Ruminating means going over the same old worries and concerns and issues in your mind, again and again – the word is derived from what cows do when they are chewing the cud. That says it all! Ruminating is most common at night when you are trying to get to sleep; ruminating is the enemy of a good night's rest.

There is a well-researched strategy to help you with sleeplessness, based on two simple notions. First, your bed and your bedroom should be associated only with sleeping. While in bed, do not sit and read, don't work on your laptop, don't have long difficult conversations with your partner. The principle is that the stimuli (feel, sight) of being in bed should be associated only with going to sleep. That leads to the second feature. If you wake up before you intended, or if you cannot immediately fall asleep, the one thing you must not do is lie there, half awake, worrying about everything that's bothering you or what has to be done the next day. After a while you will even start ruminating about not being able to get enough sleep, and that will make it even more impossible to do so. Don't start panicking: "I need my rest; I've got to get to sleep, I'll be exhausted in the morning if I don't get my sleep." What you have to do instead, is get up, get out of bed, go to another room, and do something else (read, play a boring computer game on nighttime settings, listen to relaxing music) until you begin to feel sleepy. Then go back to bed and try again to fall asleep – if you can't, repeat the same procedure.

Relaxation

There are two techniques that have become popular in psychology because they are simple to learn and easy to do. One is called deep muscle relaxation or progressive muscle relaxation. It involves deliberately tensing all the different muscle groups in your body, holding that tension for a moment, and then deliberately letting go and trying to let go deeper and deeper, feeling all the tension in the muscle fading away. When you start this you will be surprised at how often you find yourself with clenched jaw, tense shoulders, wrinkled brow, even when you don't feel tense at all. The beauty of this technique is you can do much of it while sitting in your parked car, in the doctor's waiting room, on the phone to your family, and so on. It is easy to access audio or video tapes more fully explaining progressive muscle relaxation – you will find a good one at the end of this chapter. If you do 20 minutes of these exercises as practice a few times a week, you will learn how to drop into a greater state of relaxation easily, even when you are not lying down or on your own.

A second useful technique is similar but involves only passive relaxation. Developed by Mark Schwartz and Stephen Haynes, it promotes tension release without any physical effort. The advantage of this is that some persons should not be tensing muscles as part of relaxation because tensing can aggravate certain symptoms such as pain, and other muscle tension related symptoms. The program is easy to follow and is available either as an audiocassette or a CD (see resources at the end of this chapter).

Imagery and Meditation

Another good way to increase your relaxation is to have a vivid fantasy that is calming. You could imagine yourself as a leaf floating down a little stream, just gently floating along, carried by the babbling brook. Or you could think of yourself lying in a hammock between two palm trees, listening to the sound of the ocean and feeling the warm sun on your body, enjoying the light breeze of trade winds. Vivid fantasies in which you feel safe, and in which you can imagine all the related sensations, can be a helpful antidote to painful worrying thoughts flooding into your mind. This is similar to daydreaming, but the images you conjure up must be positive.

Meditation is another activity that has waxed and waned in popularity over the years, in many different forms. There is a great deal of scientific evidence that despite a certain amount of hype, those who practice meditation regularly can learn how to become very relaxed. Invest in a couple of yoga mats to combine meditation and yoga and learn such techniques as controlled breathing. You will easily find videos on YouTube to give you some initial training. And clearly this is something you can do with your partner, so it has that advantage as well. Here the goal is not to have a rich array of thoughts like positive daydreams, but to have as few as possible – creating a "calm-mind" by emptying it of worrying thoughts. If you love to listen to your favorite soothing music, that might be the easiest of all strategies to implement.

Yoga and meditation have their origins in Zen Buddhism practices, but if you are a member of another religious faith you'll find activities that are similar. Quiet contemplation has been practiced by Catholic monks and nuns for centuries. Your church may have a regular prayer meeting. Of course the goals and purpose of religious practices are not focused on relaxation, but they can often have that added benefit.

Acceptance and Mindfulness

There are two other exercises that have become popular in recent years in clinical psychology, and these are acceptance and mindfulness training. People struggling with negative feelings and fearful, anxious, or depressing thoughts devote a lot of mental energy to avoiding or escaping these thoughts. They make you uncomfortable, so you want to get rid of them. But in fighting them off, you're actually making them worse – you're paying too much attention to them, trying too hard. The analogy is often made of someone who is stuck in a deep hole and trying to dig themselves out. The harder you dig, the more the sides of the hole collapse around you and you will never get out that way. "Stop digging!" a counselor might tell you. "Stop struggling! Thoughts are just thoughts; they are not reflections of the truth."

This is slightly different from Beck's CBT approach, which discourages only irrational thoughts. The "acceptance" approach encourages you to actually accept all thoughts but makes it clear all of them are just thoughts. Don't fight them. Accept them as having nothing to do with your situation. But that's not the same as giving in to them, because at the same time you have to do things, to act, to change your life in meaningful ways, and start doing the things that reflect your values and the kind of life you and she wish to live. Of course, it's easier said than done! You might try to remember the old Alcoholics Anonymous maxim: change the things you can change, accept the things you cannot change, and have the wisdom to tell the difference. And in Buddhist philosophy there is a focus on self-compassion: be kind to yourself, and not self-critical of you faults.

If you think these sorts of ideas might appeal to you, there are many good sources of self-help readings that can tell you more about this kind of approach. But there is one self-help idea we think is really valuable and simple to do. It is to encourage you to increase your "mindfulness."

Mindfulness involves a purposeful concentration on sensations and thoughts and experience in general, without judging these to be good or bad. The notion was popularized by an American scientist called Jon Kabat-Zinn, who was strongly influenced by a Vietnamese Zen Buddhist monk. Two important components of mindfulness are: paying attention to your immediate experience, and being open, having a sort of curiosity to what you are experiencing, and accepting it.

One of the easiest sorts of mindfulness exercise is the concept of "savoring." It is fun to start off by doing this with a favorite beverage or even your morning cornflakes. Often we eat and drink without paying much attention to the taste and flavors of what we are consuming, worrying distractedly about other things, bolting your breakfast down so you won't miss the bus, listening to bad news on the radio, or deep in conversation with someone else. To start, try to identify the tastes and texture of something you are consuming. Then you can get more proficient at concentrating on your environment, noticing amusing things, seeing beauty in a building for the first time, enjoying the details of religious or cultural ceremonies, or feeling the smoothness of carved wood. Try really focusing on your partner's smiles. Take her photo on your cell phone and later savor it – look at it deeply, look at her eyes, the corners of her mouth. Is she smiling in a totally joyful way or is there some underlying tension, a little bitter-sweetness?

Accessing Resources

Thus far we have been talking about the burdens you as a caregiver might experience while helping someone you care about. Whenever we talk about burdens, however, we have to talk about the other side of the coin: the resources available to you to help you cope with them. As more and more medical services have come to understand the need, many of them offer a variety of resources to you. Find out if they have a group-counseling experience led by a qualified mental health provider, a one-off information evening, or maybe a weekly regular meeting with other partners in the same boat. Don't be tempted to dismiss these kinds of experiences because you think you are strong and resourceful and don't need them. When your partner has breast cancer and needs you at your best, that is the very time attending sessions such as these can help both of you.

We also know the younger the woman with breast cancer is, the more likely it is you and she will need mutual support – she will have special concerns about her young children, likely be struggling with finances, and have had a shorter time to gain confidence about the strength of your commitment to her. As we discussed in Chapter 13, late-stage breast cancer is another time of great support needs, for her and you. Women diagnosed with metastatic breast cancer (MBC) are dealing with the practicalities and unknowns of a serious state of affairs. She will be looking to you for total moral support and unconditional love. And remember, it is not how much support you know you are offering – what counts is how she perceives this support. It is crucial you listen to her requests and ask her to be straight with you regarding her needs, as she sees them.

Call in the Reinforcements

Not all of the pressures of caregiving should fall on your shoulders alone. When talking to men and women who have been the primary caregiver for a woman with breast cancer, one of the most useful things they told us is about the value of asking other people to sometimes take over your role for a short while. Obviously, this will be discussed with her first, as she's likely to have opinions of who she would be comfortable with as your stand-in, back-up, or reserve team. Someone close to her, like her mother, adult child, or close friend could be the perfect relief person. But once this is decided, there's a good chance she'll find it truly pleasurable to have some other support a little different from your own.

Caregivers have told us that at first they felt guilty asking others to help, but the relief experienced of a day off or even an hour's break was considerable. And interestingly, their partners felt especially pleased by the clear evidence there were so many other people who cared for them and who were willing to help out. It has proved to be a highly positive experience all around. Identify specific actions you want your friends and relatives to take when you call on them, like filling in for you during her appointments or chemotherapy sessions so you can take a break. Identify those who will offer you practical support in addition to empathy and love. Know the people who will give you tangible aid and service when you need it most. Decide who are the people you can count on to offer objective advice and accurate information. Trust those friends who will be honest with you and provide meaningful feedback. Then too, be forgiving to the friends who seemed unable to be close to you both during her cancer but who want to continue their relationship with you in the future.

A second approach to calling for reinforcements is making use of professional resources. Throughout this chapter we have hinted that as a primary caregiver, you could be getting depressed about your depression, or anxious about your anxiety, or panicking you won't be able to cope. These can become self-fulfilling prophecies. But some of the things we have been describing are not easily dealt with on your own. Serious difficulties with sleep, or depression, or obsessive worry about your partner's illness, require professional intervention. Your doctor will probably recommend medication (sleep medicine, painkillers, anti-depressants). These can be useful, but there is always the risk of overdependence. Instead, your doctor may refer you to a psychologist or other mental health expert. If your health service has a mental health team or counseling services, don't hesitate to use them. We are confident they will agree many of our suggestions. However, the addition of a face-to-face, caring professional person encouraging you to implement suggestions such as these can help you deal more effectively with what is happening to you and her.

Trust Your Own Inner Strengths

A team of health experts and psychologists in Brazil conducted a systematic review of the many studies on the experiences of male spouses of women with breast cancer. They concluded the diagnosis of breast cancer changes the lives of everyone involved, but the feelings of loss, mutilation, indifference, and dependence are strongly counter-influenced by hope, support, resilience, and renewed energy and activities which enhance and give new meaning to life. Getting good information, accepting new responsibilities, and maturing (personal growth) were all important for achieving positive outcomes and coping.

Men and women partners of women with breast cancer often report personal growth experiences, even at a time when life seems so dissatisfying. Personal development and relationship enhancements are so worthwhile they are the sorts of gains you can strive to achieve. Naturally, we talk about resilience and coping – all things designed to minimize the psychological harm of the stress of caregiving in these circumstances. But we could look at the part of the glass which is half full. Instead of thinking of coping as ways of countering negative experiences, we can think of coping as striving to attain new learning, new awareness of the beauty of life and the complexity of wellness. Strategies such as being more mindful, trusting in your own instincts, being more accepting, are all methods that aren't simply for fighting the bad thoughts and the negative feelings. They're also for drawing on deep, positive thoughts and good, warm, loving feelings.

Summary and Recommendations

• *Adopt a problem-focused coping strategy.* Identify the issues you are facing and come up with solutions. If you have children, get them to help using the family problem solving meetings described in Chapter 12.

- *Learn techniques for relaxation and stress-reduction.* Practice having a calm-mind; do active things to stop ruminating. Decide if your catastrophizing and other negative thoughts are actually rational and accurate. Don't struggle against unpleasant feelings – instead, use them to motivate you to make active changes in daily routines.
- *Use all the resources available to you.* There are online programs, support groups, and interventions to support partners of women with breast cancer.
- *Socialize with friends as a way of having fun, not just as a way of soliciting support.* With your friends, don't allow too much time for complaining, grumbling, or obsessive talking about her breast cancer. You can be open about your feelings but try to make sure your friends and social support network think of solutions, not commiserations. Talk about other positive aspects of your lives.
- *Use additional resources.* Encouragement from others is good and fundamental to our emotional and mental stability; practical help from others is sometimes even better.
- *Use mindfulness tactics that allow you to savor and accept things as they are,* so you can focus on the good and the wholesome rather than wallow in self-pity and despair.
- *Remember your partner with breast cancer is not a saint, can't be expected always to be courageous, and can sometimes not be rational.* That's her right. You are allowed to be critical but only to the extent it is for her benefit. Hostile or snide comments and insensitivity to her feelings need to be recognized as your weakness.
- *Exercise regularly* – it is good for just about everything bothersome in life. You don't need a gym or weights or a yoga class or a personal trainer, valuable as these are – just move!
- *Recognize that anxiety, suspiciousness, depression, avoidance of feelings, and irritability (or anger) are all natural reactions to stress.* Rather than trying to suppress them or pretending you don't experience these emotions and feeling, practice positive alternatives.

Sources for More Information

https://www.youtube.com/watch?v=1nZEdqcGVzo
(How to do progressive muscle relaxation)
https://www.youtube.com/watch?v=86HUcX8ZtAk. (This video allows
    you to practice along with soothing music and images.)
http://www.guilford.com/books/Passive-Muscle-Relaxation/Schwartz
    Haynes/9781606230367
(How to do passive muscle relaxation.)

https://www.youtube.com/watch?v=wi2Q_7C1OfM
https://www.youtube.com/watch?v=AsqZRXq1kQw
(How to do mindful meditation and acceptance.)
https://www.youtube.com/watch?v=vjKltKKSur8
(Leaves on a stream – an exercise to help you separate yourself from your thoughts.)
https://www.youtube.com/watch?v=vU1-S3LgzC0
(Self-compassion – learn how to face your flaws with love and courage)
https://www.youtube.com/watch?v=ZE7VuWH0S18&feature=emb_logo
(This video reflects the hope experience of male spouses of women with breast cancer. It was funded by Canadian Breast Cancer Foundation - Prairies/NWT.)

Duggleby, W., Thomas, J., Montford, K. S., Thomas, R., Nekolaichuk, C., Ghosh, S., … Tonkin, K. (2015). Transitions of male partners of women with breast cancer: Hope, guilt, and quality of life. Oncology Nursing Forum, 42, 141–143.

Lopes, V. B., Lobo, A. P. A., Da Silva, G. B., Melo, A. K., Lamboglia, C. G., & da Silva, A. B. (2018). The experience of male spouses in the context of breast cancer: A systematic review of the literature. Psychology, Health & Medicine, 23, 89–98.

Index